1978

Living with Mysterious Epilepsy

BOOKS BY
WALTER C. ALVAREZ, M.D.

THE MECHANICS OF THE DIGESTIVE TRACT: Paul Hoeber, 1922; Second Edition, 1928
NERVOUS INDIGESTION: Paul Hoeber, 1930; translated into Spanish and Catalan
DISEASES OF THE DIGESTIVE TRACT: Chapters 2 and 4; Oxford Medicine, 1933
AN INTRODUCTION TO GASTROENTEROLOGY: Paul Hoeber, 1940; 2 editions
NERVOUSNESS, INDIGESTION AND PAIN: Paul Hoeber, 1943; published also in Great Britain, 1956; paperback edition, Collier Books, 1962
THE NEUROSES: W. B. Saunders, 1951, 1952, 1953, 1955, 1964; translated into Spanish
DANGER SIGNALS: Follett, 1953
LIVE AT PEACE WITH YOUR NERVES: Prentice-Hall, Inc., 1958; translated into 11 different languages; paperback edition, Award Books
PRACTICAL LEADS TO PUZZLING DIAGNOSES: Lippincott, 1958
MINDS THAT CAME BACK: Lippincott, 1961
THE INCURABLE PHYSICIAN, An Autobiography: Prentice-Hall, Inc., 1963; translated into German
LITTLE STROKES: Lippincott, 1966
NERVES IN COLLISION: Pyramid Publishers, 1972

Dr. Alvarez has also written many chapters and introductions for several books, plus over a thousand articles and editorials.

Living with Mysterious Epilepsy

My 48-Year Victory Over Fear
by Ruth C. Adam

Edited, with an Introduction by
Walter C. Alvarez, M.D.

An Exposition-Banner Book
EXPOSITION PRESS   NEW YORK

First Edition

© 1974 by Walter C. Alvarez, M.D.

Library of Congress Catalog Card Number: 73-92057
ISBN 0-682-47906-3

Manufactured in the United States of America

Introduction

Here is a book by a fine trained nurse who for the first forty-eight years of her life suffered terribly from many nervous symptoms, such as a violent temper, brief spells of confusion, an inability to get along peaceably with people, horrible nightmares, and frightening hallucinations. No one of the many doctors who had studied her problem had suspected what was wrong. When I noticed that her muscles tended to go into spasm, I gave her Dilantin, a quieting drug, and overnight she felt like a new woman.

Later, with my help she wrote this book, with the great hope that the story of her sufferings and her great relief from them would enable perhaps a few million persons with her nervous disease to get well. It certainly could bring health to a few million people if they could only read of her sufferings and say to themselves, "Why, I have most of the symptoms that Ruth had." Then they could take Dilantin, and perhaps be almost well overnight, as she became almost well.

She wrote this book at my suggestion when she told me that on three occasions she had attempted suicide, and she was afraid she would attempt it again unless I could teach her to do something that would make her life seem worth living, preferably something that would help many people. When I suggested that each week or so she would write me about her sufferings, and I would put that information into a book that might help millions, she leaped at the idea, and in her remaining years she wrote me a few hundred letters. These letters my secretaries, Dorothy Burnstein and Carolyn Osborn, copied, and I put together into this book. It can give readers an excellent picture of the sufferings and weird experiences of a person with Ruth's type of illness.

5

True to her promise, she never again attempted suicide, but kept thinking happily of the possibility that she could help a few million people. I am satisfied that this book of hers is the best ever written by a non-convulsive epileptic.

Why was I so willing to labor much to produce and edit this book? Because in 1908, I read a book which was greatly to influence my life and my thinking. Written by Clifford Beers, it is one of the world's great books—*A Mind That Found Itself* (Doubleday, revised edition, 1948). In it Beers told of his sufferings during the years he spent in two mental hospitals. I became so greatly impressed with what I learned from him about the strange workings of a psychotic mind, such as caused him to behave as he did, that ever since, in the last 64 years, I have been collecting and studying autobiographies of people who suffered mentally or physically in some one of many ways. So far I have collected some 875 such books, and I have given them to my good friends in the great Mayo Clinic library.

Abstracts of sixty-five of the best of these life stories that I have found are in my book *Minds That Came Back* (Lippincott, Philadelphia, 1961). The stories told by three very able epileptics—Margiad Evans, Dostoevsky and Van Gogh—taught me much about the many odd, weird, and distressing symptoms which some epileptics have, even when, as commonly happens, they have few or no convulsions. I cannot remember ever having heard in medical school a word about the dozens of very annoying or frightening symptoms that torture those millions of epileptics who never had their disease recognized for what it was—because they had no convulsions. Without a history of "fits" their diagnosis was practically always "just nerves," or "There's nothing the matter with you." Recently I wrote a book, *Nerves in Collision* (Pyramid House, New York), based on the histories of 274 people who did not complain of convulsions, and in not a single case had the correct diagnosis been made.

What has distressed me is that most of my brother physicians were taught, as I was, that "epilepsy is convulsions." Actually, the great Hippocrates, who wrote 400 years before Christ, told about non-convulsive epilepsy. England's probably greatest neurologist, Dr. J. Hughlings Jackson, around 1890, wrote enough about non-convulsive epilepsy to fill two big volumes. He knew the symptoms well if only because his cousin-wife had them. He wrote that he was not much interested in convulsive epilepsy: that was "too simple." He loved to write in detail about the many very common, but rarely recognized mild types of the disease. Dr. Jackson said sadly that he did not expect ever to have what he wrote noticed or quoted or accepted during his lifetime; and he was so right.

Dr. William Lennox, during his days the world's leading expert on epilepsy, in his two big volumes (published in 1960), had three chapters on the milder forms of epilepsy. That great epileptologist, my dear good friend Professor Frederic Gibbs, impressed me much when he told me that for every epileptic he sees with convulsions, he sees ten without them. In 1932, the eminent Harvard professor, Dr. Stanley Cobb, agreed heartily with Dr. Gibbs, saying that for every epileptic he saw with convulsions he saw many without. A number of able neurologists have written much about epileptic abdominal pains, the "borderlands of epilepsy," or those thousands of epileptics whose main symptom is a violent temper. And yet occasionally I will read a recently published article or book on epilepsy by some neurologist who does not seem ever to have heard of the non-convulsive types of the disease. He certainly did not mention them in his article or book.

What has now caused me to dedicate the remainder of my life to the helping of non-convulsive epileptics—getting them to understand what is wrong with them, and how easily they might get great relief in a few hours, is the fact that if there are a million easily recognizable epileptics in America (the officials of the National Epilepsy Society recently said that there are four million) then if Professors Gibbs and Cobb are right—and I feel sure they are—there must be, walking around in America, with their severe illness unrecognized, several million unhappy people, most of whom could be made more comfortable overnight. Those unfortunates could so easily be helped. Already, with Dilantin (diphenylhydantoin), I have given back health to some 400 of my patients, none of whom came to me complaining of convulsions; they came to me usually because they had abdominal discomfort or pain. Dr. M. T. Moore has published a dozen or more articles on epileptic abdominal pain.

Often the diagnosis is so ridiculously easy that one can make it in a few minutes. For instance, in the case of Ruth, the fine woman of 48 who wrote the letters that went into the making of this book—she had consulted many psychiatrists and had received an enormous amount of futile psychotherapy, shock treatments, etc. None of her physicians appeared ever to have suspected epilepsy. A few minutes after the woman sat down in my consulting room and told me of common epileptic symptoms, like spells of violent temper, of great fear, of confusion, depression, or hallucination, I was suspecting that she was an epileptic. Then I noticed a twitching of one arm and one thigh, and I felt pretty sure of the diagnosis. Next, I asked her if she had ever had brief 30-second spells when she was not completely conscious (petit mal, or minor epilepsy), and she said, "Sure; I have had those spells ever since I was six." Then I was sure she was an epileptic. I got electroencephalograms made on her, but apparently her lesion was so low in the brain that it did not show irregularities in the records made from the top of her skull. Then I got electro-encephalograms made on her mentally retarded brother, and they were typically epileptic; also I learned that another brother was insane, two nieces had had serious mental troubles, and another brother had been "difficult" and alcoholic. Her father and her maternal grandmother had had violent, possibly epileptic tempers.

When I put Ruth on Dilantin, an anti-convulsive drug, she quickly lost much of her great distress, while more of it came under control. Unfortunately, at times she did not take full dosage of the drug, and then some of her old symptoms would come back.

In the next nine years, Ruth must have sent me several hundred long-hand letters. Some of them were typed years ago by my secretary, Dorothy Burnstein, but the great majority were typed recently by Carolyn Osborn, my assistant, who had to learn to read Ruth's often weird handwriting. Carolyn and I then went through the manuscript, removing, as I said above, many of the repetitious and unessential stories of what Ruth's acquaintances or employers had said or done. I have used in this book only the most informative and interesting parts of Ruth's many letters. Here and there Carolyn and I have added an explanatory note that will help the reader to understand why Ruth said what she said. Often she would contradict herself or say something bitter, but as she realized, she was two persons, one kind and friendly, and generous, and the other easily angered and with a violent temper. She said she hated this second personality of hers. At times she said how lonely she was, and next day she might say how she had no desire for friendships. She tells of her frequent violent dealings with her brothers and sisters.

Ruth's father had Ruth's terrible temper, plus a tendency to fugues, in which, without saying goodbye, he every so often would disappear—for some weeks—and desert his family. Some epileptics do this sort of thing. Ruth hated her father because of his temper, and the fact that once he beat her black and blue. Her mother was kind to her, but her mother's mother had a terrible temper. Because her home was so unhappy, and she was not allowed ever to bring schoolmates to the home, Ruth early ran away to live with two grandparents; but soon she hated them for their religious severity, and so again she ran away. At nineteen she entered a school for the training of nurses. She never had a normal girl's life, with a happy home, beaus, parties and dances, and that must have had a bad effect on her. As a devout Catholic, she loved to go into the empty cathedral to pray, but because of her violent hatred of orders to do anything, she never joined the church.

A physical handicap that Ruth had was a high blood pressure which shot up when she became angry. When she first came to see me she had already had a little stroke (see my book *Little Strokes,* published by Lippincott, Philadelphia, 1966) that had left her with a clumsy and somewhat numb left arm and hand. The abnormal blood pressure kept her from ever becoming perfectly well. Also, as I said above, what kept her suffering more than necessary was her tendency to keep trying to get by without taking much, if any, of her medicine.

The most hopeful feature in her case was the wonderful change for the better in her life that came when she took the Dilantin regularly. Then she became much calmer; her temper came under control, she was less fearful; she could come close emotionally to her relatives; also she could more often sleep in a dark room, she could go on a vacation, she could go into an elevator, and she might even have several weeks of really good health.

If Ruth were here, I am sure she would be saying to all readers of this book, "If you see that you have a number of symptoms like mine, beg your doctor first to send you for electroencephalograms, and then ask him to give you four capsules of Dilantin (100 mg.) a day, and see what it does for your nerves. Sometimes it helps much to take with each capsule a half-grain tablet of Mebaral." The results then are often excellent. With mildly epileptic "problem children" I often have gotten perfect results with a medicine called Deaner (deanol).

I hope readers will not be too shocked at Ruth's stories of her wild rages. As I said above, the important point is that, as she often said to me, "I have two people in me, one hot-tempered, fiercely independent, scrappy, and quickly enraged if anyone tries to order me about. I will never be a 'human door-mat.'"

Sometimes, like other violent-tempered patients I have known, Ruth would go into towering rages even when she was alone in her room. She would then curse violently and perhaps pound the wall with her fists. But as she said, "There is the other half of me which is full of kindness. If a beggar asks me for a quarter, I am tempted to give him all the money in my purse. The good side of me much dislikes the bad side, and I am ashamed of that side. Every so often I will change so suddenly from my good side to my bad side that I will fear I am going insane."

The reader who knows all this about Ruth will be less likely to judge her badly when she tells of having flown into a rage. Incidentally, she hated the day or two of fatigue that followed a tantrum, and sometimes she remembered in time my warning that she would have to pay heavily in fatigue for having indulged in an angry blow-up. Also, readers will now understand why in one letter Ruth will say she is happy to live alone, and in the next letter she may say that she much wants a home and children and (rarely) even a husband. On one page she will tell of cursing like a pirate, and on the next page she will tell how deeply religious she was, and how sure always that God was taking good care of her. What happened was that she had changed suddenly from one of her natures to the other.

As I have said, Ruth always deeply resented anyone's effort to *order* her about. She even resented it if a physician told her to come back after a week, or "ordered" her to follow a certain regimen. She said she was happy because my two assistants and I never gave her any orders; as a result, we never had anything but courtesy, kindness, trustfulness, and great friendliness from her. Because she could not stand being ordered about by a hospital head nurse, a year after I first saw her she gave up nursing and eventually became a housekeeper for some well-to-do people with two children.

Only twice, for a short time, did Ruth feel love for a man. One man was one of her psychiatrists. But nothing came of it. When she wrote him an affectionate letter, he did not answer. For a short while she roomed with a fine woman for whom she had some affection, but soon she could not stand that. Evidently there was no lesbian type of affection between the two.

Ruth so loved little children that she would gladly have had some born to her, but she could not stand the idea of having a husband, and also she was afraid that any child of hers might inherit her types of suffering. Two men in succession offered to keep her in an apartment as a mistress, but she immediately turned them down. As she said, she not only could not give love, she could not accept it when it was offered her. She could not even receive a small gift from anyone without feeling demeaned. Once when her nice employer gave her a wristwatch, this so enraged her feelings of independence that she either gave it back or threw it away. One of her nieces was apparently similarly outraged when Ruth sent her a generous check as a graduation present.

At times she would do curious things. For instance, when her mother died, Ruth burned all the family pictures. When she left her work as a nurse, she destroyed all the letters she had ever received, also all the addresses and telephone numbers of the friends she had made in the nursing school.

Ruth's letters are full of statements to the effect that she wished she was dead. Even with the great improvement in her health produced by Dilantin, she was often tired and fed up with suffering and loneliness and feelings of "what's the use?"

In November, 1964, Ruth had a stroke which produced much difficulty in talking and swallowing. Naturally, she became depressed and tired, but bravely she kept doing some housework. Until the last week she kept writing the letters to me. Her health kept failing, and she died on April 1, 1965.

She so wanted to help other brain-injured people that from her small salary she saved some $2,500, which she willed to the Brain Research Foundation of Chicago. She got a lot of satisfaction from knowing that her savings would someday be used to help other people like her to get well.

As I said, she also was full of hope that this book telling of her sufferings and the help she got from Dilantin, would bring hope and good health to thousands of people who are now suffering much as she suffered, especially during her first 48 years.

I must emphasize here that the person who reads this book, and notes that he or she has many of Ruth's symptoms, may not have true epilepsy. He or she may have only what the great British neurologist Dr. Gowers, called "The Borderlands of Epilepsy." Unfortunately many people so hate that awful word "epilepsy" that they would rather go on suffering than take an anti-epileptic medicine that overnight could take away their distresses.

Actually, there should be no disgrace in having epilepsy. As the great Hippocrates used to say, in 400 B.C., it is a disease of the brain just like any other; it is certainly not due to any god or devil. No one is ashamed of having a brain tumor, but if the tumor should cause convulsions, the patient would be terribly ashamed.

The great shame associated with the word epilepsy is due to the fact that in the Bible we read that Christ cured epileptics by ordering a devil out of them. I have a copy of an English Bible published in A.D. 1500 which contains pictures showing Christ standing in front of an epileptic, out of whose mouth is coming a little black devil. It is sad that this acceptance by Christ of the ancient idea that indwelling devils and gods produce diseases should still—nearly 2,000 years later—be causing millions of good, innocent people to feel greatly disgraced, and to endure much mental suffering.

Let us all now try to fight this unjustifiable idea that epilepsy is shameful. I can never forget a time when I was being registered in a hotel and the bellboy who was to show me to my room crashed to the floor as if his legs had been kicked out from under him. He lay there unconscious for half an hour. My only feeling about his behavior was that of great sympathy. This feeling became greater when I heard that the young man had planned to marry next day. I never heard if he did marry.

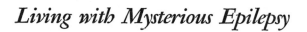

Living with Mysterious Epilepsy

Chapter I—1956

In February, 1956, Ruth wrote to say that when she came to me she was desperate, fearing that any day she might wind up in a mental hospital. She kept wondering what was the basic cause of her spells of twitching and jerking. She knew that the spells were more likely to come when she was worried and nervously upset, with her mind jumping constantly from one subject to another, and with a desire to run far away and hide.

In her first letter, Ruth wrote: "I prayed for guidance, and the answer was, 'Go and ask for help.' So I made my decision to come to you. I first went to church to pray, and as I sat and watched the priest at the altar, and the people kneeling in prayer, tears ran down my cheeks. I prayed too, and suddenly I felt calm and the burden was lifted. With the peace and hope I felt, I knew I could talk to you. But as I sat in your reception room, I became so worried and frightened that I nearly got up and ran away. Happily, when you walked in and smiled at me, I relaxed. I smiled back at you, and for the first time in my life I was not afraid of a doctor. Soon I realized, as I sat across from you, that you had me pretty well sized up."

2-6-56   Thank you for letting me pay my bill. [DOCTORS OFTEN DO NOT CHARGE NURSES, BUT RUTH HAD SUCH AN INTENSE DESIRE FOR INDEPENDENCE THAT SHE MADE IT CLEAR THAT IT WAS IMPORTANT TO HER THAT I ALLOW HER TO PAY FOR HER VISITS. TYPICALLY, SHE SAID, "I can't ever stand being dependent, and having too much pride is one of my faults." HER RESENTMENT OF ANY KIND OF OBLIGATION, EVEN OF GRATITUDE, IS SEEN CONSTANTLY IN HER RELATIONSHIPS WITH PEOPLE;

LATER WE WILL READ HOW SHE BECAME ANGRY WHEN HER BOSS GAVE HER A WATCH, AND SHE THREW IT AWAY. EVEN THE RESTRAINT OF BED-CLOTHES DISTRESSED HER, AND AS WE SHALL SEE, SHE PREFERRED TO SLEEP IN THE NUDE.

I HAVE FOUND WITH MANY PATIENTS, AS WITH RUTH, THAT MY TELLING THEM THE TRUTH ABOUT THEIR ILLNESS, EVEN IF THE TRUTH IS DISTRESSING, BRINGS THEM PEACE OF MIND, AND COMFORT.]

3-3-56　　　I am keeping notes and watching my moods before and after taking Dilantin. I was able to be calm on duty in the hospital until an aide made a nasty remark. Thank God I was able to keep quiet, but I was boiling with rage, and trembling as I walked away; my chest felt tight.

3-4-56　　　I am still angry today, but calmer. On duty I felt a wild impulse to harm someone. [MANY PEOPLE LIKE RUTH, WITH NON-CONVULSIVE EPILEPSY, HAVE TOLD ME OF THESE SUDDEN IMPULSES TO INJURE OR HARM OR EVEN KILL SOMEONE. THIS FRIGHTENS AND DISTRESSES THEM. "SOMETHING INSIDE OF THEM" TELLS THEM TO KILL A NEARBY CHILD, OR AN OLD WOMAN.] I prayed for self-control. These impulses keep trying to come back, but now often I can control them. For a while, fear is gone.

Last night, I was almost asleep when I had the beginning of a convulsion. My face started to jerk, also my right arm and upper part of my body. There came a blinding light, and then elephants started walking by, and horrible bloody faces of men appeared. I put my light on, and took another capsule of Dilantin. I heard voices talking until I fell asleep. [THESE WERE HALLUCINATIONS OF SOUND AND SIGHT.]

3-7-56　　　As I sat talking with a friend, my mind warned me to expect a convulsion. I just sat quietly and willed that nothing would happen. And it didn't. In the past two days I have been quiet, alert, and have had none of the old slight periods of forgetfulness. [PROBABLY PETIT MAL.] I now wait quietly for traffic lights to change. [OFTEN RUTH, AT A STREET CORNER, WOULD CROSS AGAINST THE LIGHT, SAYING, "What the hell: I don't mind death." THERE WAS ALSO AN ELEMENT OF HER RESENT- MENT AGAINST BEING "TOLD WHAT TO DO" BY THE TRAFFIC.] At times I forget everything; I find myself standing in the middle of the street, or in the rain without an umbrella, and how I got there, I don't know.

Since taking Dilantin, I am no longer afraid to go to meals with other people. [FORMERLY, SHE COULD NOT STAND TO BE AT TABLE WITH ANYONE ELSE; SHE ALWAYS ATE ALONE.] My voice is quieter, and I speak more slowly; I don't feel I have to be on the go continuously, though I like to walk after lunch. I have lost my fear of being out of a job. I always feared tomorrow and next year.

3-8-56   I keep dropping medicine tops and knocking over bottles that I reach for. My head and right arm jerk slightly at unexpected times. I want to do many things at once. But after taking a Dilantin capsule, the impulse to scream or to swear over some slight mishap is gone. I don't stumble in my room as I did formerly, and I am much neater.

3-11-56   My electric iron burned out, but I kept very calm and used a small iron I had; no swearing! My right arm is jumping slightly at frequent intervals; my head turns quickly, without any reason. I am dizzy at times. I have a strange feeling of being two minds at one time. I want to care for the patients carefully, and yet deep in my mind I feel like saying to the head nurse, "Stop asking for so many things to be done; please remember that I am human and have to get moments in which to breathe."

3-12-56   On my day off, at last I was able to go up in a crowded elevator; I could step into it! I felt bad as the elevator started down, but I was all right. It has taken me weeks to get up the courage to walk down a darkened aisle in a movie house. [THESE SMALL DAILY PROBLEMS THAT RUTH HAD HAD TO FACE FOR A LIFETIME WERE VERY DISTRESSING TO HER, AND, FORTUNATELY, THEY WERE MUCH LESSENED BY DILANTIN.]

How often I was afraid of being given shock treatments. Sometimes I felt drugged, and I must have screamed. I had a hallucination of a nurse with hate and madness blazing behind her glasses, and I seemed to see and feel her hands on my throat. I heard her say, "You will be quiet." I was unconscious after that.

Now, *after I take Dilantin* I find myself being nice; a woman at peace, doing things with less fear. Some fears still rise in my mind, but for hours I feel the quieting effect of the drug, and I am always humming or singing to myself.

3-16-56   I made up my mind in childhood to belong to myself [THIS WAS RUTH'S CONSTANT THEME.] I'll give to each person their due, but some part of myself I will keep to enjoy—like my life when I am off duty.

3-18-56   My left arm and hand jumped and struck a cup of coffee. Of late this has been unusual—most of my trouble is in my right hand and arm. For some reason, I am very nervous before I have a day off. With the help of Dilantin, I could drink coffee continuously. I do not now have to sit on my nerves as I did in the past. When someone gets angry I can stop and see two sides of a problem. I will look out for myself when necessary, but I won't have any more attacks of anger if I see one coming on. I hate arguments, but I am always ready to stand up and answer back. *Without Dilantin to keep me calmed down I could not go on.*

3-20-56   Soon I'll start looking for another job. I just walked into a home and asked about a position for employment. That was something I formerly wanted to do but could not face up to. Taking Dilantin seems to help the walls of fear to fall before they build up. I am ashamed to pray so much, but often I do so.

3-24-56   Dilantin keeps me from being foolish, walking out on a job, or arguing with the head nurse. Alone in my room I swear a little, but the old awful tension is gone. Last night I was able to get on a darkened elevator (the light was out); I had a slight fear, but I went in. I am now able to sleep in the dark; for years I could not do this; the darkness terrified me.

4-10-56   Last night after I turned out the light, I was conscious, but dozing, and sinking into a very deep darkness. The face of a man appeared, very sad in appearance. I had no fear as I saw him; I felt my body stiffen and there was a jerking; I felt a slight impulse to scream, but was quiet. As the attack ended, I felt fine; and putting on the light, I went back to sleep. I woke this morning with a throbbing headache; I felt as if my head would burst.

4-14-56   I had an argument with two people today; I stood my ground but I acted calmly. I trembled with rage and felt like walking out, but I did not run away. I have an appointment for a new position Monday. This time I want to go back to being a nurse; but I still prefer to let someone else worry about washing the dishes.

I woke at 2 A.M., with a severe pain in my ankle; my foot was turned up. I wonder if I had a convulsion? My mind was jumping with many questions. Later I cried, and felt relieved.

4-16-56   I was dozing this morning, early, and felt the onset of a convulsion. This time my head kept jerking back. I felt I was sinking into deep darkness. Then in my mind I saw deep black clouds shot with rays of gold, and deep black eyes that barely appeared as dots of light. This attack hardly let up when I had about eight lesser attacks. The eighth one was severe, and I moaned once. All through this I was conscious; I could open my eyes as attacks ended, and all looked clear. I have taken a Dilantin capsule [PROBABLY SHE SHOULD HAVE TAKEN THE FOUR I PRESCRIBED], but I still feel that more attacks will follow. This is the first time I can ever remember a morning attack. *Any argument causes me trouble a day or two later.* [RUTH HAD TO LEARN THAT FOR AN ANGRY SPELL SHE HAD TO PAY A HIGH PRICE WITH SOME SICKNESS.]

4-17-56   I am definitely back in the world of people, and I refuse to give in to fears.

6-29-56   I started the new drug to add to Dilantin [Mebaral, ½ grain]. In about an hour, a reaction started—a staggering walk, a pressure in my chest and arm, left side. Nausea. I was frightened, and decided the best thing to do was to give up all medical care; also to disappear, and die in peace. Common sense returned and I laughed. I realized I need help, and it's silly to be afraid.

I went to bed about 10 P.M. I fell asleep, then woke up in my dark room and saw five women standing by my bed, holding a meeting. I joined the meeting. I had no fear, but some time in the night I screamed in my light sleep. No one heard me.

I had to be on duty at 7 A.M. I had nausea, and staggered as I walked. On duty I was fine; I watched carefully as I lifted a child, to be sure of my balance.

6-30-56   In bed, in the darkened room, last night, as I started to fall asleep I heard voices of Chinese people; a man stood near me; and I seemed to be in India; his eyes were so black. I opened my eyes and fell asleep. Later I heard a child calling for help, and I realized it was a sound within my mind. Later, the child appeared to be laughing, and at play.

7-9-56   Several times I have been very close to tears; I cry occasionally, when alone, for no reason. Then I feel better; very happy and carefree. My hands are steady, but for a tiny second I can't spell a single word, or I feel overstimulated. As I write a letter, my mind outraces my hands. At times to add or subtract a single amount for my budget leaves me confused.

At present I feel wonderful, and I don't get tired. When I go off duty I go to the beach. I can walk slowly and my mind is calm.

7-10-56   I went downtown, and everyone was friendly and kind. With the medicines I am on, I don't have the shy feeling that it's wrong to buy something nice. I stopped to buy dishes to entertain a niece or an occasional friend. Now when the Muzak plays gay music, I want to dance instead of walking sedately down the hall. *The medicine stimulates my happy feelings.* I find it's best to take it on duty when I am feeling guilty; then with it I like my work.

Interestingly, *now after using Dilantin, at last I can accept a kiss from my favorite brother.* I never could stand family life. And loud laughter and loud talk. My greatest joy in the hospital is caring for two spastic children. The little ones are getting used to me, and I am learning how to care for them. Dr. Alvarez, you healed me with your wonderful truth and kindness. It is best that I remain a nurse. *I love the wonder of seeing pain eased, and hope building back someone's mind.* It's a great job. A few minutes with a child is such a joy.

These medicines you gave me knocked the walls down between me and the world. [THIS SHOWS RUTH'S POETIC NATURE.] I now walk from work two blocks to the hotel in which I live, and I love every minute of it. Even at night now I am not afraid. Before I came to you, with a walk in the dark, I would have died from fear. Now, on duty, I can go all over the hospital in the dark; I can stand quietly and finish one task at a time. My mind is beginning to organize each task.

Now I am beginning to relax. I can enjoy a meal with the radio on. I no longer have to behave like an old maid or a bitter woman. I try to plan sensibly ahead in developing hobbies that will help others. Now I save dimes for books; I feel so rich. The glory of standing alone on the beach, water touching my shoes. The sunset and soft winds. I try to face life with courage and hope. *I used to be so afraid to laugh and relax.* I always put it away for tomorrow or later. [IT IS REMARKABLE HOW MANY AREAS OF RUTH'S LIFE WERE CHANGED AND MADE BETTER BY DILANTIN.]

I am responding to life and its wonderful gifts. This medicine works so strangely. I am making new friends. A very fine and wonderful man at Wilmette and I enjoyed making life brighter with laughter. He was always showing me some article in the newspaper about women and our ways; he had such a wonderful kindness and insight. He was a bachelor 80 years young in heart. If one may have love instead of affection, we had it. There are so many meanings to the great gift of love.

I took a capsule and fell asleep, and my mind raced, making pictures like something turning. The night clerk told me I sleep quietly now [A REMARKABLE DESCRIPTION OF WHAT DILANTIN CAN DO FOR AN EPILEPTIC]. Your Dilantin has let down the bars of fear; I work alone on duty, trusted, and without the old anger, I can ask for advice or discussion any time. This is heaven. I couldn't stand it before, day after day, people saying, "Do it just so." But with this medicine I find I am conforming to routine without pressure. The fear, the rush, is held down. I no longer feel the desire to be overtalkative; I can plan my work, and now people are coming into my life. Soon I'll be serving a cup of tea or coffee to my friends, and we can talk. Formerly I was so afraid to be warm and alive. I eat breakfast happily now as I never did before. I laugh and joke, but I am serious.

On Dilantin, I am starting to talk less quickly. [AN-OTHER PATIENT, WITH SYMPTOMS LIKE RUTH'S, COMPLAINED MAINLY OF SUCH RAPID SPEECH THAT PEOPLE COULD NOT UNDERSTAND HER. THE DILANTIN HELPED HER GREATLY.] Also, I am able to be courteous and I don't have to be constantly on guard and on duty about my emotions—anger, fear, and tension. On duty I now sing to myself, and nobody laughs. And I sang out loud on the street. Everybody is kind to me.

7-21-56   In talking, there still sometimes is a slight break; suddenly for a tiny second I forget everything. My hands now grasp objects more steadily, and I am organizing tasks better. In caring for patients I am relaxed. I am getting less talkative, but there are still tiny seconds of "not being present" [petit mal]. I can now see my problem and I work carefully and as calmly as possible.

A night clerk in the hotel told me he heard me screaming and crying in my sleep. I never knew I did that. Now he says I am quiet. I was very angry one evening; and I did lots of screaming in my room. When I went off medicine, faces got distorted and out of focus, and vision blurred.

I am swearing a little more than usual, but I am better than in the past. I felt panicky the other day about getting on and off a crowded elevator; but I made it.

8-2-56   I had a wonderful day; I started my vacation. My mind is working calmly. I find a smile, and acting a little dependent makes everybody want to help me. I really love fun.

9-25-56   In bed at 9 P.M. Some time later I had a strange feeling that I would have a convulsion; suddenly, clouds of darkness seemed to envelop me, and a frightening face tried to pierce these clouds. I felt fear, nausea, and an impulse to scream. My whole body was jerking; the spell didn't last too long. Then slight tremors came in different parts of my body. [FORTUNATELY, RUTH'S JERKINGS USUALLY CAME AT NIGHT.]

All day at work I wonder if I'm doing right? Does each patient and child get the understanding and kindness he should have? At times I want to disappear, but I know the job must be done, and I have to prove to myself I have the courage and insight to do it.

10-4-56   As I fell asleep last night the mental pictures were a series of bright spinning objects and nightmare faces, but no more jerkings. *When anything upsets me, I am a nervous wreck for a long time.*

11-23-56   On three separate days, I have had a close brush with death. I had the gas range on; the window was open, and wind caused the fire to flare up high. I carelessly reached over the fire and closed the window in my usual hurry. I felt quite warm and jumped back. I was wearing a nylon uniform that I always starch a little; I think that caused me not to get on fire.

The second time I was tired and sleepy and hungry when I got home from duty. I heated food on the gas range; in turning the range off I couldn't see how to cut off the flame; I turned the gas back on without the flame, and nearly killed myself. After eating a meal I sat down to read a book. I was lost in that book when suddenly I smelled gas quite strong. The room must have been half filled with gas. Quickly I opened the window and turned off the gas, and went back to reading my book. On my way home I crossed a street, and barely made the curb as a speeding car dashed by.

12-15-56   Today, suddenly, as I looked at the floor, a face appeared with black, burning eyes. This face brought to mind an unusual experience that I have been afraid to think of or talk about. I think I was then under medical care for high blood pressure. I worked in a children's home some years back, and at the time there was much controversy about starting a union, which caused many arguments that upset me. One night in a hall, suddenly all was dark; I remember standing still, frightened, and knowing I must not scream. The wall I faced was covered with what I thought were grapevines, and through these vines, hundreds of black piercing eyes glared at me. How long it lasted, I don't know. Then the hall light was burning again, as usual. I pulled myself together and decided I was on the verge of a bad breakdown. I buried the experience deep in my mind and never spoke about it. It was some three months before I was over my fear of that hallway.

I was afraid to tell my doctor about this experience and the spasms I had occasionally. He had become annoyed with me at one time about something I had mentioned; I could never remember what set him off, but he went into a rage! And so I picked up my coat and started to leave. He said, "No; I will tell you why I want to let you go." Later, he repented and tried honestly and sincerely to help me. I tried at times to tell him I was afraid of being scolded. He knew my fear of the dark, and any time I was fluoroscoped he kindly took my hand to reassure me. I felt in a dark room that I had to get out and far away.

I remember the first time I became afraid of the dark. In a hospital I had to take a just dead child to the morgue. As I walked in there the light was on, but suddenly it went out. Outside of the door I heard giggling. I stood quietly because I didn't want anyone to know I was sick with fright. The light then turned on and I left. Years later, a classmate told me who the nurses were who had played this joke on me. For a long time after that I could not stand being in the dark alone.

My childhood had been a world of terror. School days

were with an old maid teacher whom I hated. My grand-parents never seemed to see any good or happiness in me. The teasing of my classmates made going to school an agony for me. There is one strange happening I can never figure out. At times I have felt the coming of death, and events later have shown I was right. Recently, I had a night of extreme restlessness. I felt that someone I knew was dying; I could not get rid of this feeling. Then my classmate wrote me that her father had passed away. Another time I got the idea that soon I would be deathly ill, and, sure enough, I soon was. Fortunately, I recovered; my brother telephoned me to say that while at sea, he had felt that I needed him.

Chapter II—1957

1-2-57   At present, after taking Dilantin and Mebaral, my old habit of swearing has stopped. However in my apartment I often mutter plenty to myself under my breath. When I want to swear on duty, I go to the bathroom and lock the door; there is a nice corner there where I can let off steam. Tiny children sense one's moods; hence with them I try to be calm and relaxed.

1-4-57   I had a problem in a restaurant today; after drinking coffee I picked up my change, but suddenly all became blurred. I was "not there." The waitress gave me my change and handed me my wallet.

1-7-57   I went very close to death twice, when I didn't want to live. I remember the night I decided never to trust anyone again; I decided to work hard and never know what friendship or kindness would mean to me. Thank you for your trust in me.

1-10-57   The night nurse told me I am crazy, and my work is poorly arranged. I just kept calm. Why argue with an old woman?

1-12-57   I am afraid of the night nurse. She wants to provoke me into a fight and I refuse. I know now that if I am to keep good health, I must learn to live and adjust myself to all personalities.

For the past two evenings, I have felt close to tears—very nervous and afraid I'll never get work done or give the children in the hospital enough attention. Tonight, as I talked with a patient, a hallucination appeared. I saw an immense set of dentures dangling from fine wires. I went home as soon as I could. I know now I must learn to accept problems, responsibilities, and especially, to get along with people.

Women will always be trying to make me over. I know nothing about men.

2-6-57   People like me can't talk to just any doctor. But when you came in and smiled in a way that made me feel I had been guided by God to you, at last I was able to speak and ask questions. [THIS STATEMENT SHOULD ENCOURAGE MANY YOUNG DOCTORS ALWAYS TO BE FRIENDLY WITH PATIENTS AND TO BE SURE TO SMILE AT THEM.]

On the streetcar, I talked with a woman who was depressed; she couldn't find a job. So I told her about employment agencies, improving one's appearance, and putting on a smile; and I told her to forget the burdens she once had. I said, "We women that are alone are foolish; we hide in a world of fear; no one cares about us. But there is no law against being attractive. It's fun to be alone, save money, travel, and go to church. Start with a prayer, and think what you can be thankful for."

On duty, at all times now I guard my speech and my walking. Last evening I couldn't remember the names of patients, or of the relief nurse. When I carry a child, I am careful to stay close to a wall, up against which, in case of dizziness, I could lean. Also I walk slowly through a door, so that I won't bump myself. Since taking Dilantin, I am getting fewer cuts and bruises; I am not falling over so many objects, and I am turning on the hot water tap more carefully. I wake up smiling, and am glad to see a new day. How often in the past I prayed to die, and never to see the dawn.

I have started reading newspapers. For a while, I couldn't do that. But I still have a fear that I may not have enough food to eat. Occasionally in the day, or at night when I waken, I have a feeling that a presence is close to me. A man seems to stand and watch, a mocking smile on his face. I don't feel fear, but how often I have turned suddenly to see who is near.

Now I know that fear is a prison, and that bars can be broken with your help.

I remember that once, when I worked in a home for unmarried mothers, there was a girl of 15, and for some reason, nobody had a kind word about the child. The hospital staff said her attacks of fainting were an act; and no one had seen such a frail child, beset by a thousand fears. I asked to have her spend a day downtown with me. We had a lovely day, but as we walked and talked, all became dark for me; I heard a voice say, "She will die."

I was friendly with this child, and stood up for her defense often. When she came back, six weeks later, I received a call to see her; the nurse was hysterical and said the child was putting on an act. I ran to her room and found her on the floor. I picked her up and took care of her.

2-9-57   Yesterday, while at the stove preparing lunch, I must have had a spell of petit mal, because I came to, to find the package in my hands on fire. [RUTH HAD MANY SUCH ACCIDENTS, DUE PROBABLY TO SPELLS OF PETIT MAL WHICH ARE NOT ALWAYS CONTROLLED WITH DILANTIN.]

When a patient told me I am a happy-go-lucky type, with not a care in the world, I thought, "I'm not a bad actress."

RUTH'S EARLIEST MEMORIES

[THESE ARE RUTH'S EARLIEST MEMORIES, SOME THAT HER MOTHER TOLD HER ABOUT.]

I was the second child. The first child was a boy who soon died. [MANY CHILDREN WITH A POOR NERVOUS INHERITANCE DIE IN INFANCY.] I weighed 2 lbs., 13 oz., and at first I was thought to be dying. My father upset my mother by going into a rage because he had wanted a son and not a daughter. The doctor and my father almost came to blows. I don't know at what age I started to have spasms. Mother said I was not an easy child to care for.

An early memory I have is playing with a mirror, and through the reflection trying to walk into what appeared to be another room (like Alice in Wonderland). I can remember once seeing mother unconscious, seated on a chair. One day, Mother gave birth to a beautiful blond boy. My brother and I climbed into Mother's bed to be hugged closely.

In my childhood often in a rage I scratched my face with my hands until the blood ran; and pits were made in my face. I hate my grandparents today just as I did when I was a child. Once when we had no food, Grandmother was angry because I cried. My mother borrowed money in order to buy bread.

At school, I was a good student, but I was always restless; I hated to be quiet. Once the teacher put me in a dark closet, and forgot me there. I cried, and finally fell asleep. That is one reason why for years I had much fear of the dark. I was always nervous and jumpy after that. Often as a child I was just as dirty and devilish as I could be.

When Mother came home with a new baby boy, I was disappointed not to have a sister. But I learned to love the boy. I cried and asked my father why I wasn't a boy; he said there was nothing to be done about that, and I would have to be happy as a girl. [THIS EARLY DESIRE TO BE A BOY MAY HELP EXPLAIN WHY RUTH WAS USUALLY ASEXUAL.]

My father and mother were short-tempered. I had invited some boys to my house for a tea party. When my father came home he angrily sent the boys out. With this I became very angry, and father beat me terribly. With that, a raging hate filled me, and I told myself, "I'll never marry." I hate men and always will. [RUTH KEPT TO HER RESOLVE AND NEVER MARRIED OR EVEN HAD A BEAU.]

In my girlhood I often had to take care of my brothers. Today, as I look back at the years past, I wish they had never been born. For some reason we avoided our blond brother, although he was handsome, with long golden curls and gentle, loving ways. Brother E., with lovely black curly hair, was everybody's pet. I always comforted him when he cried.

Eventually we left the town where I had been born. We tried many places. The farther my father could take us from a city, the better he liked it. I had only two and a half years of high school. I couldn't make the grade because I seemed to be going blind, and so I left school. How awful, that I was afraid to tell my mother I couldn't see well. I had headaches. Finally, I got glasses, and then I saw a new world. But I hated high school because I made no friends. Also, often I could not find my way around the halls so I would go into the wrong room and the teacher there would be annoyed with me. Never afterward did I live comfortably in the world of people. My childhood had been so unhappy.

When I was nineteen I went into three years of nurse's training. I worked hard, long hours; I had many worries; and I was glad when I graduated. Then my mother died of tuberculosis, and my father and I grew ever more bitter towards each other. We were ready to kill each other. Already I had hell's own temper; and how I raved. Often, after a rage I would feel drained and ill. How often death seemed to me the best way out.

Please forgive me, Doctor . . . I can't go on now; while writing this I have cried so much that I am tired; I can't cry any more; so goodbye.

You asked me if I now have any friends. Actually, I have two friends, both nurses. One was my classmate. *I make some friends, but I never keep them.* I hate a life cluttered with people, I still fight against having people in my life. *I prefer to be alone.*

I'll try, after I am calmer, to continue this letter to you.

2-10-57   A TERRIBLE NIGHTMARE. I have passed my first big test in a year—a nightmare that seemed very real. After it, because I seemed to have seen real people, I searched my apartment carefully—under the bed and furniture. My windows were well closed, and coal dust on the sills had not been disturbed. I had gone to bed, and was restless: later, when I was half sleeping, there came the horrible nightmare. Suddenly, I felt a hand on the bedcovers, pressing onto my hip. My hand grasped the foreign hand, but I couldn't move it. I held on; I wanted to scream, but couldn't. My mind said, "If this is real, how did the person get in?" Suddenly, I fainted and sank into waves of darkness. When I woke, I lay quietly for a few minutes, but when I saw no one was around, I got up and checked the apartment.

Now as I write, I feel calm. I won't tell anyone except my classmate about this, and I may not tell her. I still strongly suspect that someone really was in my bedroom. The only way anyone could enter my room would be through the window at the foot of my bed. I have now decided to keep two lights on when I sleep. Also a street light shines into my room.

2-14-57   *I can't ever thank you enough for the help your medicine gives me.* Each time now I get ready to explode, I ask myself, "Why do that?" But still at times I feel like a volcano ready to erupt. Then were I to blow up I would destroy all I have gained in mental discipline. I am over the shock of that awful nightmare. For two days I slept with a light on. Now I am sleeping in the dark except for the street light which shines into my room. With that I feel calm. So I am beginning to feel that the awful event I went through was probably only a hallucination. If anyone was in my room, it's all over. And should he be there, next time I might as well try to have courage enough to see how handsome my unknown visitor is. The worst that can happen will be my death.

[LATER.] Recently, when I went for a vacation to Jasper Park Lodge in Canada, I had a nice quiet time. But a strange woman followed me and said she had been watching me. She said I impressed her as a woman proud, yet humble (that I have been told once before); we walked and talked. She asked me to write some articles about the strange events in my life. And she gave me a book. She said her daughter was a writer.

When I got back, I did a lot of thinking and praying. I don't trust strangers, even when they think I do. I felt that only *you* have the right to ask questions. So I have never written to her. I have no desire to have more than the two friends I now have.

Long ago, when I went to my psychiatrist, often my body was present, sitting apparently calm, listening to what he said. But actually, my mind was having a wonderful time, taking me into a nice, quiet park. To me, the psychiatrist's conversation was a lot of rot. But I don't want to escape when I see you. I promised myself to be a good patient with you, and to behave.

2-20-57 I was too shy to tell you, but recently I put myself on a diet. I am using common sense and eating all the basic foods to stay well. I decided *that* 48 *years* is no reason to be overweight. I stay about 110 lbs., more or less.

I have now decided that what is past is over. I now laugh more often. Now it's time to look back at the world of fear, and these are the events of childhood I have started to remember. When going to school, some of the older schoolgirls tried to take my clothes off. How I cried and fought with them. The fact that I was afraid to tell my parents about their behavior tells much about my parents.

I shall never forget when I was a child in the first grade; my parents were so angry with me that they said they would give me to some woman they knew. They told her I was bad. I was stunned. I didn't like the woman when she looked at me. I wondered: did my parents love me at all? To this day, when I think of that cruelty, tears come to my eyes. *Mother said I was always afraid to have my picture taken.*

As memories crowd, back come the tears. I am now glad to be alone.

2-26-57 Today I have two scalded hands to show for a second off guard. I turned on the hot water faucet and somehow both hands remained for some seconds under the boiling water. My hands jumped when I felt the burn. The swearing I then did was out of this world. If I see the devil shaking with laughter, I'll know it was a good show. As usual, I cried enough from anger to need a sheet to wipe away my tears. Then I laughed at so much raving and exploding. Aren't I funny?

I walked to the lake, and listened to the roar and rush of the waves, as I walked along the shore; I asked myself, "Why the fear? Why the hate and worry?" I have no answer, but often when life looks like darkness, I burst out laughing.

I can write only as I see my life and the fears I fight. Anyone who thinks I am a timid angel had better look at me once more. Yesterday I answered someone back, and it was a pleasure to do so. I was so boiling with rage I could have cried. I know deeply and sincerely that when I am out of this nursing job, there will be no more of it for me. Last night when I finally got off duty, I exercised the usual privilege of a woman. I did a good job of swearing and crying. I went to bed and prayed that I would never live to see a new dawn.

I half woke to find myself having a nightmare. I felt a tiny body lying across my chest. I held a tiny hand and the other hand was sticking something sharp into the back of my head. I was awake enough to realize it was time to take action. I moved my head, sat up, and felt fine.

Now I have decided always I will keep calm and relaxed. Why should I get so upset? So what, if I get thrown out of work? I'll never be a martyr, and won't be anyone's whipping boy. All the years of my life have been full of tension and fear. *Now I am going to laugh and enjoy what time is left.*

I have always made a point never to save any letters. I am now trying to go back into the past, to write down more of the memories of all the past years. At the present time I cannot. I slammed a mental door shut, and now I feel terror in trying to open it!

3-1-57   My day off—and at home I really let my temper explode. I talked out loud, and did plenty of swearing and raving. I went to bed, and as I closed my eyes, in the darkness, I saw hideous people who started to walk past in review. Slight twitches suggested the onset of spasms.

3-3-57   This is a remark you made when I first saw you: "Go ahead; you can tell me anything." I laughed. Then I knew I could. The relief of your not fussing about my blood pressure: I could be me, the patient, and not a guilty prisoner of fate.

I have seen Alaska in the quiet beauty I dreamed about. I'll start a vacation fund; what's money put away but for a purpose?

What a wonderful change, Doctor, you have wrought in me. At last someone understands the fires I burn with. I thank you deeply and sincerely. I feel wonderful. Now at last I am going home to visit my family. I never dared visit them before when I was in a stormy mood. And regardless of how angry I get, I'll try to use more common sense in the hospital when on duty. A child on the floor heard me get angry on duty and he was upset. I am distressed to think I could let a helpless child hear me get angry.

I save up all my tensions until my day off. Then heaven have mercy on me. What a week I have just gone through. While I was walking past a hot pipe, my arm jumped, I got a burn, and that set me off like an atom bomb. For some reason, even when I am calm, the sound of church bells drives me wild. There is a harshness about them that I can't understand. *I want quiet so bad that I could cover my head and hide in a dark corner.* If I am ever found dead, I ask myself, will the cause have been temper or an accident? I would like my work better if only I could feel more warmth and kindness in the hospital. People, children—all need that wonderful feeling of love. If we only paused to think, how much time is there on earth; death is permanent—or is it?

I walk as often as I can to the beach, to the beauty of the lake; and often I am tempted to say, "To hell with life." Plenty of places into which to disappear. But this time I can think and keep calm. I do have to laugh even when I am crying for being so dumb.

Once for a year before I went to a psychiatrist, *I fought a battle against suicide.* But now I can't go against the promise I made to you before God—that I will never try again to take my own life.

3-8-57   Never again will I wish anyone to go to hell and stay there. Sometimes I wonder what kind of woman I am. Of late it has been peace, and as I sit and try to collect my thoughts, I am afraid to look back at the world of fear in which I used to walk.

My two youngest brothers went to sea. A. left home at 22, able to walk and talk, and to try to live without me; E. left home at 18. They knew my lamp burned always in the window for them. A year went by, and finally I left the hospital and did nursing exclusively for a woman doctor whom I had met when I was managing a nursing home. She asked me to take her cases. I would be on 24-hour duty. Often when I left, after the patient recovered, I would be in bed at least a week, drained of all life. Recreation—I never knew the meaning of that word.

I rented a small apartment. My father and I did not see each other after my youngest brother left home. I wanted to be alone, to read books, to walk endless miles. My nights alone, I slept as little as possible; I was afraid of my awful nightmares.

Well, my life crashed at long last, with the memories that have seared and burned like a living flame in my mind for years, I came off a case numb; suicide was the only way out. I didn't smile any more, and I walked in a daze. My job was done. I straightened up my apartment and planned to die about 3 A.M. The doctor called me for another case about midnight; and I refused to go; I said I was worn out. I think she knew what I was planning. I shall never forget that cold winter night. Before her call I stood and looked at the stars, so cold and far away, and I seemed to die. My emotions were frozen. From that day on I was to walk in a world of fear and distrust; I feared that never again would I trust anyone; I would give myself only to the sick and helpless. Nobody would ever again have the chance to hurt me.

Later, I sold everything in my apartment. Then I spent three months working in a small hospital. I had only two friends, one of them my classmate who is to me a sister, and very dear. I got a position in a hospital. I heard many questions and stories about my being cold and unfriendly, but that didn't trouble me.

The war came, and I was sick with worry about my two younger brothers, one in the Army and one in the Merchant Marine. No news about them for months. I stopped reading newspapers. I saw as little of the other nurses as politely possible. And finally I knew I couldn't go on. So I went to a psychiatrist. To this day I ask myself, "What was he talking about?"

I can't go on—my mind feels blank, and I am as afraid at this moment as I was in the times when I was put under anesthesia. I'll gladly tell you anything, but I can't write now; *I am too afraid to look back.* I remember the awful attacks of wanting to scream while eating meals with other people around. I cannot write now—I am afraid.

3-25-57   An attack of anger left me with the usual problems of poor sleep and shaking hands. I am having trouble holding any objects in my hands. After four hours I want to get out at night and never stop walking.

3-28-57   [INTERESTING BREAKS IN THOUGHT: THE FOLLOWING IS TYPICAL OF PEOPLE LIKE RUTH.] For the past two days, I am having trouble remembering anything I asked for on duty or in a store. But I am improving all the time, and these breaks in thought are something I must accept and try to conquer. My trouble on the morning shift in the hospital is fear. When someone comes along and raises the roof about the way I do something, instead of following a schedule, day after day, I can't stand it, and since I am no angel, I wish deeply and sincerely that my head nurse would some day face as great a fear as I do; and I don't feel guilty. I can't honestly say I am sorry. Often in the past I have wished that bad luck would strike down someone who had hurt me. A patient once said that there were days when my eyes looked like those of an angel, and other times they looked like those of a devil. She was so right. I live in two worlds; often I am trying to subdue the bad half of me and to be good. That is one reason why I walk alone, and make no friends.

One day on duty I couldn't use the correct words to make

a sentence; I was confused, and my thoughts were mixed up like a crossword puzzle before it's worked out.

7-21-57   Some people who have trouble come and tell me of it. I suffer worse, if possible, than the person who is in trouble. About two weeks ago I got into an elated mood; I have been very dizzy since, and at times I could argue with the devil. I am damned if this job will lick me.

I talked to a wonderful man who is happy and contented with his life. His grandchild was ill; he had a month's vacation, and all his wife wants to do is be around the child. Well, life has taught me one lesson. Any woman that has raised her family should look out, and go on a vacation with a wonderful husband. There is something sad when a man like my acquaintance has to come to the beach alone; we had a wonderful talk.

People like myself, as you know, are ready to run faster than to stay put. Here at home, about once a week I go off like an atom bomb. Occasionally *I hear voices, but now, since I know it is my brain acting up, I don't worry.*

7-22-57   *Now I am looking over the second year of treatment and what it has DONE FOR ME. I NO LONGER FEEL LIKE WALKING CONSTANTLY AT NIGHT, AND I AWAKE calm and smiling. When I get hell from an overwrought head nurse, I am quiet.*

My trouble is that at times I am too easy a mark; tell me a hard luck story and I want to give you my bank account, clothes and everything. Often people tell me they wish they had everything, from health to a bank account. I just laugh, but to me, life is a battle each day.

I can't believe all men mean to harm one. Often at the beach or when traveling, I talk with strange men. I could never be happy married. *If I married and something deep in my mind should cry out for freedom, immediately I would have to leave husband and the house.*

How often in the past, after raving at my brothers, I walked miles. I love the beach when there are few people there. Silence to me is a healing balm. Living away from the world of women is best for me.

I wish you could see little Miss Two-and-a-Half Years Old, at prayertime, with her little hands folded, her little head bowed and her pair of beautiful blue eyes. They gaze into mine. The children relax and listen as I stand and pray. I am no angel, but a child's greatest need is not the fear of death and hell.

When nurses hand me a line about loving nursing, they are damned bigger liars than I am.

7-26-57 In *The Three Faces of Eve,* which you suggested I read, I saw myself. I, too, am a woman whose mood changes, sometimes making me feel loud, noisy, overly talkative, overly friendly; but I am lucky. I never have a severe headache before these mood changes, as Eve did.

7-27-57 This was my day to get up early. I was up at 6 A.M.; I just had to get out. I went to the beach. On the pier I met a lone fisherman. We had a wonderful, quiet talk, and exchanged ideas and views. But I was in my calm, nice mood.

I remember the day I came to you—I was so afraid, I felt so mentally ill, my hands were so jumpy. What would become of me? Cancer? What difference would it make; I wanted only to die. I felt you were the only doctor who could help me. How did I know that? Long ago I read an article by you, and I wanted to write you, but I couldn't; how did one dare to write out of one's loneliness and fear? I still rave and swear, but not so often; I still usually stay out of the lives of my brothers and sisters.

It's the most wonderful thing that happened to me. I can be helped to lead a useful life. I can now talk with men without being self-conscious, and something deep in my mind warns me when to be on guard.

The man on the pier said, "You have a wonderful way of seeing life: a kindness. You look nice." I like to wear slacks for a walk, but makeup and looking feminine is a must for me. I really enjoy being a woman. Today I am not writing clearly or thinking clearly. I keep feeling I am going out mentally.

Last night, at 11 P.M., as I was walking home something made me turn quickly, and I saw a man following me. I wasn't afraid, but hell's flaming fires flared in me. Had he dared to come close, I would have killed him by striking him on the head with the flashlight I had. I was in a wild rage. For him to follow me! I had not flirted with him, so I was not at fault. I got home safe, and took medicine. Partly undressed, I sat in my armchair, and began to have slight tremors. I saw darkness lit by a lovely picture of willows along a stream, then lights, then a hallucinatory picture. But I sat still and it passed.

I now feel emotionally a change in me. I do things that may be pathetic to others. There are times when I am worried: will I suddenly someday disappear and find myself married to someone, or lost and alone in a strange place, my family afraid I am dead? Will I let go of all control and get to raving so much that a mental hospital is the only place for me? Am I as a patient too dependent on you for mental help? I worry sometimes. But I made up my mind to walk alone, and now I find myself looking over my shoulder like a child to see if you are there. In the back of my mind, I worry about things that may never happen. Can I ever be taken off Dilantin and Mebaral completely?

To me this is silly, but I'll tell you about it; as I write I see flies on this box or flying around me, just one or two; but I doubt if there are flies anywhere. Is this a hallucination? I see misspelled words in my letter, but I feel O.K. [THIS IS SOME RAPID-CHANGE WRITING DONE WHEN RUTH'S BRAIN WAS NOT WORKING WELL.] The headache is easing. Life is a battle; one day at a time. Well, you met the guy; is fighting; and I'll eat a good lunch. I won't be a blockhead and starve my nerves. I see the letters I make, the words I can't spell. I'll try to be careful and put a clamp on my mind.

Today I want so much to laugh I might laugh at a funeral. Sometimes I wonder, where have I been? What happened to me? And like the slight lifting of a mist a memory starts to waken, and then I know that time is running out.

7-29-57   Today my mind burns to talk, to take shut-ins and the dear people through the door called imagination. Mental television is fine, as long as one comes back to live normally. Now I am looking at my future. God brought me so far, but He is also showing me this: to be a woman is a great and wonderful privilege!

7-29-57   [LETTER FROM RUTH TO A FRIEND] Dear Gertrude: Take my hand, dearest sister, and again let's walk together, into the beautiful world that today we call imagination. I hear your sweet words, spoken with tears, "An understanding heart." I walked out yesterday, and saw a little bird; my heart flew in prayer with him. I read a book the other day about an Indian tribe; they always caught and caged a wild bird as they buried their dead, and then the bird was released, so the spirit of the departed could go up and up with it.

I hear church bells, as I am resting and dozing. A darling bride is going into the church, and when the ceremony is over and everybody gathers on the steps, pictures taken, the bells peal so joyously. Being a woman, and sentimental, I run for a box of Kleenex. So what. We can peek, can't we? A sincere prayer for the best and loveliest life for the tiny ship that sails out on the ocean called matrimony.

Now we—you, brother and I—are going to learn to dance. First, I'll practice this new art, or is it an old one, called GETTING ALONG WITH MEN. And being shy, as you and I are, just let me handle the details. I don't want just anybody to teach us to dance. Let's decide who we like best and INSIST on that person.

When I dropped something recently I did not get angry. I have an idea the Devil sat back and said very sadly, *"Boys, it's no use; she is getting to be a good woman!"*

Recently we had in the hospital a very handsome man belonging to a religious order; so handsome that in spite of the Good Book and its teaching, I had a conversation with him.

7-30-57 The Devil nudged me, I know. And does there breathe a woman so emotionally dead that she doesn't flirt a wee bit? What did I get? A beautiful lecture about God and the Devil.

What am I doing? Trying to be the woman I should be, with guidance and help. I am passing on to you these words my doctor spoke to me one day: "Each day is a battle that must be fought."

7-31-57 My youngest brother told me some years back: "You never let us grow up. To you we are still 11 and 13 years old." Well, I am trying to talk now to my brothers as men. How can I blame them, when for years they put up with my fear, my nightmares, and my attempted suicides? They deserve plenty of credit. During my last visit to the doctor I had since 1947, I could tell from his veiled remarks that he considered my brother and me "mental cases." My youngest brother has gone to psychiatrists, in the Army and out of it, to find out why his legs ache so.

My younger brothers both asked me to come and live with

them. But not me. I was too frightened ever to sleep without a light, and also I kept walking the floor night after night, working myself into a nervous exhaustion. I have lived so long in the world of being damned independent, preferring death to help; how could anyone ever help me? Now I know it isn't wrong to say, "Please help me." I admit that I need it. God spared some wonderful man a mental hell with me as a wife.

Some place in my mind I want and I crave excitement, but the medicine keeps me calm and relaxed. Sometimes I get my old sense of fear. In the past I imagined my brothers meeting all sorts of deaths. Me, who crosses the bridge that I may never see, with the storm-tossed mind that seeks escape so often. Now I refuse to run; I'll fight. But I love a storm when all the furies of hell break loose. Something wild in me then seeks escape.

Today I plan to enjoy the thrill of being 50 years old. You should see my hospital family, with all faces lit up. So I said, "Sure; we will call it the 'Mamma R. Get Younger Party.' No presents allowed."

Yesterday as I came on duty, in a chair by the door sat one of my darling make-believe sons. Of course, I got a kiss, then to the kitchen I was escorted in style to give him a drink of water, and to the youngsters in wheelchairs, kisses before work. With adults I am serious; I try deeply and sincerely to listen to such persons, and then to tell them a little story to make them laugh.

You make it possible for me to work here. Now I see myself as the person I am, and I understand the attacks of fear I get. The other day I walked far, thinking I knew where I was, but I got lost. I had to stop in a drug store to be given directions to get home. I know I looked upset. The lady behind the counter said, "You became confused." I was frightened.

Dr. Alvarez, this may be my imagination; I shall never ask; but as our first interview terminated, I felt that you said to yourself, "Now I have made the needed mental contact with this patient. From now on I will know where I stand." Before that, I was so scared I thought I had better leave, and quick. But I would not be so discourteous as to run out instead of walking out calm and relaxed. I told myself this: remember the day I came to you and got the feeling that at last I was where I belonged. Your heartwarming smile, the healing talk you had with me has been for the best. What of it if I didn't have any children; I have had many sick children in wheelchairs, putting little arms around my neck, and saying, "Mamma, do you love me?" and the goodnight kisses.

When the nurses see me taking time out to laugh with a child, and to kiss him, they sometimes laugh at me and say, "Ruth, are you crazy?" But they say it with kindness.

8-11-57   This day I felt my brain was on fire, and I wanted to rave, and talk continually. [SHE HAD A MANIC SPELL.]

Years ago, my feeble-minded brother and I were alone. He had his room, I had mine. We had neighbors that woke him up with their laughing and making remarks, when in his sleep he would run across the roof. [SLEEPWALKING IS A COMMON OCCURRENCE IN BRAIN-MALFUNC-TIONING CHILDREN.] So eventually I had him nail his window shut, and also the bathroom window so he could not go out.

Recently I dreamed that I was alone in a park at night and men started to come out from behind the trees. One grabbed me from the back and got my hands. Hell's blazing rage broke loose in me. I got myself loose, and then I slapped and ripped and tore at the man's face. The blood was streaming, but no other man came to his aid; they slunk away. I felt sorry after I hurt this man; but did I say so? Hell, no. I told him to remember this: any woman alone has the right to walk in a park at night.

I love children, and I must care for the helpless. *If I had no purpose in life, I would have nothing to live for.* A baby I fed was about to leave the hospital, and this made me happy. We all loved him. As I fed him, I cried. To me each child is special, and the children laugh and fight; and "Mamma" has learned this. Each evening the children and I have a candy party.

The other evening, all of the children were around "Mamma." We were all going on a trip, and the whirring stool at the desk was the imaginary car we traveled in. A little matter like crossing oceans, and flying—we never trouble about that. Off we went to Israel, with the children asking questions: I told them we would talk to people, meet other children; and what happened? The imaginary driver said, "Mamma, we are now in India." This is where we went: Israel, India, Japan, California, Ireland, and the North Pole. I am still tired from that supposed trip. And the youngest child was me, of course.

Once, when with a psychiatrist, I told him about my being so restless. At a dining table, I would take a paper napkin, tear it to shreds, or keep twisting the corner.

I see now, as I have talked with you, Dr. Alvarez, that I have put my hand out to touch something on your desk, but often now I can sit quiet, and my hands are quieter. This is a lovely gift of peace that you have given me. I have to be alone in a church to feel the great peace I crave. A Franciscan Friar once said he would say a mass for me and someone prayed for me. This means so much.

Strange, so much of the world I don't understand, and yet I must be ready to live in it.

8-23-57   Today I was so confused; I knew I was in a

department store, but I couldn't figure anything out. I felt I was going into a fog. Yesterday evening I was tired and cross, so I lay down and half dozed. I began to feel my body twitching and I saw a very tall, troubled young man standing, biting his fingers. I came to with a jump. The headache I had recently for 3 days was due to my having become overemotional.

8-27-57 I woke up after dreaming that my mother and I had been together. We were happy, and I woke feeling comforted. Mother said, "When the time comes, I'll come for you."

8-28-57 I get periods when I want to be quiet, and not to write anyone a letter. In these periods I get depressed.

I woke up at 4 A.M.; I lay quiet and it seemed to me *I left my body on the bed, while my mind walked out.* I seemed to be on a lovely sunlit street. My mind came back, and I was ready to take my body out of the bed. Now my mind is getting blank, and I don't know what I wanted to say.

8-29-57 The other night I was afraid to go to bed; the recent murder of a young girl had upset me. So I stayed in the hotel lobby for two hours; the night clerk took me to my room, and my fear left me.

9-1-57 Sunday I got myself into hell's own rage when I feared I was about to lose my job. At times I am ready to walk out, but then your voice I hear, saying, "Keep calm."

There are times, as you know, when I have a blank instead of a mind.

9-6-57 I heard that my elder brother, with his high blood pressure, had a heart attack. Like me, he didn't want anyone, even in the family, to know that he was ill. I didn't now, and never will, offer to nurse anyone in my family. After a while, I'll call up and find out if my brother can see me. It has been years since we have seen each other.

9-9-57 Sometimes I feel as if I am being restrained,

and as if my life had become too uninteresting. Then I want to get out of doors quick. I have to work and to enjoy what I am doing. I love the world of beauty, music, people who are not nurses, soft voices, and the peace at twilight, or sunset. You have given me a peace and comfort beyond words. You have given me so much, I'll try to behave.

I have made this decision: my sister-in-law is a strange woman; but who is perfect? I received a letter from her long ago, telling me never to write my brother. So I wrote him a nice letter at his store, saying I would like to visit for a little while, but I would stay at a hotel. So far, no answer. I am not going to drop in unless asked to.

9-16-57   If anything ever happens to me, don't be upset. At night, in my mind, I see a black panther walking in a jungle.

[WHAT RUTH WRITES HERE IS SO TYPICAL OF HER.] *I am not an easy person to know. One minute, I'll gladly walk through hell's fiery flames for someone, and the next, to hell with everybody, and I don't give a damn.*

Suddenly I don't care if I never again read a book, so I've stopped going to the library. I listen to the radio, to the news. Don't ever tell me I have to visit anyone. Movie theatres don't appeal to me; I can't stand the thought of walking into a darkened room. In the world of today, many people are racing out, striving for education and diplomas. I am just plain me. I just want a chance to give the love I have to give. [BUT NOW RUTH THINKS CURIOUSLY.] And yet it is like something asleep in my mind that stirs: a sleeping thought that is not good. I refuse to jump in the lake, and I tell myself I can't go on as I am doing.

I notice one thing: I am getting to be a good listener. People tell me about their problems. And if the problems are tragic, out comes my Kleenex. And who said a kiss and a pat on the shoulder is wrong? But of course I let the married men just talk, and I give no kisses. A pat on the hand, a tear wiped away by each of us is enough.

I seem to be the only person that behind my tears has laughter.

Doctor, you have given me more hope than you will ever know; and people like me, lost, afraid, when at long last God feels there is a job for them, they get better. Give me music, then quiet, and I don't give a damn in hell. I know this—I hold on pretty tight to the hand of God, and everybody in each religion can point out the pitfalls in my way of thinking. All I can say is, "Thank God for sleep, deep and unbroken; for waking with laughter and the joy of another day." I am not blind; I know that life can and will hold problems, but I can rave to myself, then pray after that; sit still; and I can't go anyplace any faster, anyway.

9-17-57   But I am visiting nobody in my family. Minding my own business is best; *I hate being in people's homes. I get that awful feeling of a wild thing being placed in a cage.* When I get too excited, I'll try to stay in a bath. *But doesn't anybody else ever get that awful feeling of being trapped, taking orders, having to listen?* Behind the locked door of a bathroom, I can let off a blazing volcano; then talk out like an angel, so some dear woman would wish me a husband who would carry me around in his arms all day, and give me no less than 10 or 20 children.

I bought a police whistle, but as yet I can't even get a slight noise out of it. But when I find a man following me and I am not in the mood for company, what is a hell-raising temper for? A good attack of rage, and the poor man may be looking down and saying, "I didn't do anything. She fell, and when I looked, she was dead."

Thank God, I am still able to joke and laugh, but I know that people like me are problems. Our doctors are to be pitied. We patients can be so eager to be helped, yet suddenly we will run away, trying to find an escape into darkness. *Why am I so frank with you? Because you asked me, and said I could help others.*

9-18-57   I have been boiling since my sister-in-law destroyed letters I wrote to my brother. I'll go to a lawyer and bring a damage suit. I love most my youngest brother who is feeble-minded. My two younger brothers seem to me to be like sons I never had.

Dr. Alvarez, I realize that at present I am in a period of elation from tears to laughter. I can live no one else's life. Today I laugh when people tell me I would have been a wonderful wife and mother. It is best that they don't know the truth.

I must make sure at all times that I am thinking before I move—when I am lighting the oven or the gas range, turning on a burner; I don't want anyone to think I committed suicide.

This is my hunger: to discuss books, to listen to the story of other people's travels, to get more out of life than just being a children's "mamma." Why not learn to be a convincing talker? When I was working in the home for aged people, I saw people helpless, being treated like no pedigreed dog would be. I was ready to run out of there after 3 days, but I stayed 8 months. Then I came to you just in time for help. *People should be saved from a mental life that is worse than physical death.* I found that many fine, wonderful minds have been allowed to stagnate, with nobody giving a damn about them.

Well, I had better calm down; after all, I don't wish to die while writing this.

9-19-57   This is something that has made me do a lot of thinking, and frankly, I can't forget the piercing eyes of the man that made me feel undressed. I see him as I write;

just now I am unable to spell. Perhaps this man had had one drink too many.

When these storms start in my mind, the feeling of being so elated, hell's fires rising, tears that come so easily, I tell myself, "Yes, I am saved"—because at long last I can say to a doctor that I am not the person who can stand restriction in a hospital; I can't stand being told to stay in bed when I want to go out and walk. What a relief to admit to you that I fight, each day, for what I want. At long last I try to talk slowly.

I have no place to go, and even hell, after one of my attacks of raving, doesn't seem to be opening a door, the Devil bowing and saying, "My dear, we are so pleased you made it. All of us had really given up hope that a sinner like you would become an angel."

I am beginning to enjoy meeting people, as long as I have a home to be alone in. I have to fight pain and not get twisted up like a pretzel. I am repeating something very nice my sister-in-law said in a letter. Before I came to you for help, she would never have said it. Always my family acted as if they had to worry over me. Well, here is the remark: "You are an attractive woman. If I look like you after my seventieth birthday, I will consider myself very lucky."

9-20-57   Here is the truth; you know more about me than I will ever know about myself. I have to be busy, *watching these awful storms in my mind and not showing what I am going through.* I must never let anyone see or guess when my mind is off duty. That is why I am usually outwardly calm, and relaxed, and I realize that black eyes like mine can show fires when I want to give only a sparkling look. Now I make sure when I wake up that for a while I lie quietly; *until I know if I am dreaming or awake.*

9-21-57   Last night I dreamed I was looking for a

plastic cup; I wanted to give Miss Three-year-old a drink before she went home. And I got all kinds of glasses except the one I wanted; and was I mad. Oh, no; just ready to boil. Eventually I found the cup and milk, and gave my darling her drink. But next morning I woke up boiling, blazing mad, and with a headache. [WHAT A DESCRIPTION OF WILD TEMPER.] I'll wait and see how often the Devil and I meet.

9-22-57   I realize I can say this to you: something not easy to admit to others—that at long last I am beginning to learn. I know there are medicines to help me, and they have helped. [NOW RUTH SHOWS SIGNS OF BECOMING CONFUSED AS SHE WRITES.] I am confused here, I guess —I don't know—I am in my living room, conscious, but what do I say? I feel slightly dizzy and a strange feeling. I feel as if I am going to be whirling into space. Damned if I'll give up. I'll relax and turn on the radio. Now I am back. This is my battle—never to let people know that I get confused. My classmate is the only person that knows the truth about me, and she has promised no one will ever know. I love my brothers, but I don't tell them. At first I couldn't understand that one's mind can come and go, that there can be spaces in between, so I guess I come and go, and that is what I seem to be doing now. Well, I feel better for having talked to you.

9-23-57   I seem to do my clearest thinking when I get up at 5 A.M. At other times I get depressed. It wasn't easy to adjust myself to children that can scream or get angry or smile and with their eyes tell me what they want. I have shed tears, from the exhaustion of work, and I went to bed worn out.

I am learning that regardless of physical age, I am a child, and often a bewildered one.

One day I sat down and wrote my sister-in-law a letter, and I received two lovely letters back. She said I should have been a writer. I told her about the funeral I want: lights, music, and all the trimmings, and if necessary, look in the phone book and find a minister to say a few words. Death can mean that a soul tossed around by many storms at last has found rest. And now, like water being turned off, my mind is going off; without spoken words. Now I see the heartache, the struggle, of patients who can't talk.

Now I have this fear: I wake up and feel wonderful, but I have been terrified; as soon as I get up, will someone come in? Can I dare to take a bath? What am I afraid of? It is too bad that I didn't die long ago. I am now facing, with your help, emotions that at long last I can speak of openly. What is wrong with psychiatry when so often it is nothing but a discussion of sex?

There was a woman who long ago kissed her husband good night, and I knew it was the last earthly kiss. There was the time I heard my brother call me when in danger. And there were the times I have heard in my mind, "Ruth, you are going to die," and death came pretty close. Once when I was taking a patient to the operating room, she said to me calmly, "I won't come back alive." I knew this was true before she spoke.

9-28-57   I was sitting and reading the newspaper, when suddenly I felt that my heart had stopped; my mind was a complete blank; darkness fell, and I couldn't hear my clock tick. I wanted to scream and could hear myself muttering, my face twitching; all over I felt a jerking with my whole body in motion. I had a feeling this was close to death, but I had no fear, only relief that life would be over, but still I felt I'd be damned if I would give up. My heart didn't want to beat any more; but I got over this, and soon felt my heart beating slowly and regularly.

Deep in my mind, I heard a baby cry; there was an ache in me to hold a wee one. But I am comforted; it was best not to have children. God has his reasons.

I refuse to leave this work: this is where I want to be.

9-29-57 [TYPICAL OF RUTH'S SUDDEN MARKED CHANGES OF MIND IS HER NEXT DAY'S STATEMENT.] I just quit my job. I just couldn't take it any more, with no mental stimulation in it; nothing. And I have reached the place where a job must hold more for me than day after day setting up trays, putting food on, and seeing that the children are cared for. I'm sorry—I didn't do what you asked me to do—to retire with dignity. Did that damned secretary care when she called me after 10 P.M. to try to blame me for the way a child felt? I am no angel; I could not forgive. I am so sick of nursing, I am ready to get rid of the uniforms. Then I'll just have to find something different. Why do people think nurses don't care how they live? I cannot live or work in a place where no one ever talks; a nurse is treated like she doesn't exist, and I can't stand that. So I may soon be washing windows or something; I don't know.

10-3-57 From the day you accepted me as a patient, I have seen myself undergoing a change. I have always found it better to get rid of the past. When I have to work with a damned fool who is married to her job, and thinks a nurse is dust on the floor, to hell with her. Does one have to go to hell to earn a paycheck? *A woman that can give one a look of bitter hatred—what did I ever do?* Now I feel like a woman out of prison; all I ask for is a job where there is courtesy, quiet voices, and nice people. In a place where I worked, the maid told me, "Don't speak to anyone." There was a woman there so sneaky that she stood behind doors or on the stairway to listen. If I had a patient, there she stood, like an avenging angel, looking at her watch; always checking to see if I was working full time. To hell with those conditions.

Now I have a chance to be among real people, out of the world of nursing. I hear that these people for whom I expect to work are of the intellectual type. There are two children, girls. I will have a chance to travel. So I am going out into the world. I want to learn to live with healthy people. I am willing to learn to wash windows—anything—*but I must find mental peace.* I am not ashamed to go into service. *There is nothing I want but a chance to serve others.* All right; nurses can sneer, "Ruth, a servant!" It doesn't matter to me. You, Doctor, opened a door for me so vast that I refuse to go back.

10-4-57   Today I am making an appointment to talk to a Catholic priest. For the first time in my life I am daring to reach out and say, "Father, please let me talk with you."

From the day I knew that I was accepted as your patient, I studied you and your staff, and I said to myself, "At long last I need not run any more."

I particularly want you to have some lovely Wedgwood blue vases that I have, and if you know someone that needs a radio, I'll have mine checked, to be sure it's in good condition and then I will give it. I have learned from you to burn my bridges with care.

10-6-57   I think for the first time in all my life I have stopped running and have started to think for myself. *For weeks the impulse to walk at night, to get out of the house, go out and keep on going, has disappeared.* And today I am going home to visit with one of my brothers.

I realize there is no sense in saying, "Please help me," and then trying to find a door marked escape—or suicide. I realize that some people will take me for a simple-minded child.

[THIS TELLS MUCH ABOUT RUTH.]

Recently I saw a butterfly, trying hard to get off the pavement, and so gently I got it into my hand. Then I took a stick, and Mr. Butterfly took a dainty hold. I carried him to where he was safe, and my heart flew with joy. Off he spun, so gay, over some bushes.

I don't plan to sit back and do nothing and use up all my savings; but my mind must get over the screaming of a helpless child.

10-7-57 What I expected from nursing was a job where I could grow mentally, meeting doctors. But what is it? Glorified housekeeping. Today I feel good. For the first time in all my life I am just plain, honest loafing, and enjoying it. And my mind is finding peace.

One trouble with nursing is that it spoils many women for marriage. The rules of training, such as not dating the interns; the lack of money with which to look nice, or to have pretty things. At long last I am cleaning house and giving up possessions that it's best not to keep.

I only know that for me God exists everywhere; not in four walls called a church, or a special holiday (SUNDAY) when people dress up and look grave, and then on Monday when they go out as mean as ever. I believe in freedom of mind—to really think, and not in a religion that forbids much. I am a seeker, and independent.

10-11-57 Last night I had a talk with a priest. I needed to talk with a man to be blunt. And he said that I was on the edge of a breakdown. I told him this: never, before I placed myself under a certain doctor's care and guidance, could I have come to him just to talk. My fear of the dark, the nightmares, *the continual walking until almost dawn because I was afraid to sleep*—all this is gone. I walked out of the hospital because I couldn't take any more despair, any more of such fears as people get in a hospital. I couldn't take any more people in hospital robes, with nothing to talk about but aches and pains.

I visited my family. It's better for all of them that I don't come back, because I don't belong in their life.

And I have the chance now to go into a real home, to work and see how people live. I do not want to be part of the family. Why is it wrong to be willing to scrub a floor, or to iron clothes?

The priest tried in kindness and gentleness to show me that a woman with compassion for others should be a nurse. I told him I could not go on. *The warmth, the wonderful feeling that one is doing right, has left me.* The sick and the helpless have dropped out of my life mentally, once and for all. At a nurse's meeting, hell's bells—one can find more human interest and life in a home for the aged.

This new job has done something for me; and it has all been good. I learn to live with normal people and not the sick. I want now to be where I can see people, not in uniforms or hospital gowns, but in regular clothes.

10-12-57 I have decided to frame a small picture of the Madonna and Child—a reproduction of a painting. There is something so calm and sweet in it. For a woman like myself who faces storms, a beautiful picture like that does much.

I can say this from looking women over: one either has that wonderful, warm feeling for the helpless, or one is just cold as an iceberg. Some women can't stand children. *But in the nursery, the colored women are wonderful.* Some women so hate children that their babies are picked up by one arm —which hurts.

These people I am to work for are highly cultured. With them, I feel like I am becoming a different woman.

From now on, *I REFUSE to have a convulsion; a slight one in the daytime caught me unaware,* and recently a second one tried to come, but no more; I will fight back.

10-13-57 Now, I marvel that a woman need not be aggressive, saying, "Move over, out of my way"; she can be a dear, kindly lady. I have always been one of the very lucky women—always somewhere doctors, nurses, patients tried to go beyond the wall of fear to show me that life can be lovely.

If I had a daughter, I would want her to have the best education, but also enough problems to make her think. *I have run so far there is no more place to go,* but it's amazing—today I find myself liking people. A woman like myself must have something beautiful—a symbol of faith, such as the lovely, gentle reproduction of the Madonna and Child that I treasure.

My employer asked me, "Can we depend on you to stay with us next year?" Then deep within me there was awakened a strange, restless feeling. I must conquer this restless feeling, of wanting to be on the go. Because, for me, to iron and clean are tasks I enjoy; I want now to do simple things.

10-14-57   *This is what the years have taught me: do not be afraid to confide in a man or woman—just talk and the puzzle falls into place.* I do not feel I have an aggressive attitude toward life. In all the years, I have honestly enjoyed being ME. Frankly, I often say the wrong things, but I try to be honest.

10-15-57   I get depressed, and I sit down and cry, and later I feel fine. I have had periods when I couldn't read a newspaper. I would tear up the magazine I had bought. But I have more of a sense of freedom; I feel a release. *I have parted with my possessions; and all I kept I can keep in a shoe box!* Deep down I know this: my greatest happiness can come in ministering to others. The good priest was right in this: I am, and always will be at heart a nurse. My fight must go on as long as I live.

10-16-57   When it comes to mental confusion, sometimes I still have it. I just can't make up my mind. So at first when I got a phone call about a job, I would say, "No," and I would plan to go back to nursing. But then I sensed that I can't go back to nursing because the thought of that is more than I can stand.

10-17-57 In search of a job I went to a couple of agencies, and both times walked out boiling mad. *I could not remember the street and number where I lived.* Sometimes a flaming fire tells me, "Go on." Damned if I am beaten.

10-21-57 I know that I shall never live to grow old. And when everybody is getting frightened and hysterical about the future, with the ministers and everybody screaming, it doesn't worry me. In the ancient days man dreamed; in the world of today I too dream. One can pile up earthly possessions from hell to heaven, but what is it really? Just junk. And still everybody yells for more and more. *Lovely warm memories are my jewels to treasure. And as I took your hand and pledged to write these letters, I knew suicide was out.*

There is one thing I have always wondered about. What is this strange fear of death? Some people are in such a panic. But so what; sooner or later the final hour comes to all men. As for the time when my hour comes, and I go to sleep and never wake, I have no sadness, no fears; "it is written." Many people don't know that kindness and love can bring a baby from the verge of death back to life. *And as long as some doctors try to treat physical ailments without treating also the mind, then much of their work will be useless.*

I don't know where I am going to go now, but *from the day I met you I have been alive. I try to mix, but I will never be part of the crowd.*

10-22-57 I thank the Good God—He has given me much, and I *pray that I will not have to go on too long.* My mind has awakened, but it is like a fire that is dying out, that flares up once more. But I don't care or give a damn.

10-26-57 *Now I am beginning to enjoy being alive.* I have been looking for work, but so far everybody in town seems able to do without me. But I am not worried. The problem I have is that people seem to think I am the delicate type that never knew hard work. I enjoy talking to the agents even if I don't get the job.

I shall never forget how my mother impressed on me the idea that it is not wrong to commit suicide in a case of rape. Once a man told me he had planned to attack me. I shall never forget how pale I felt myself get. But I stood straight and told him this: that if he raped me no one would ever know what had happened because we would both be dead!

10-27-57   At times I have a strange feeling that beside me walks an unseen friend.

One night when I seemed to be in a black fog, I stepped off a curb. I heard a man call me, and I got back just in time before a swiftly moving car had ended all my problems. I thought I had seen the light change at the corner.

One thing I'll never figure out. Why is it wrong to be happy, to laugh, to enjoy being alive? When I listen to a minister on the radio talking about everything being a sin —love, movies, television, and heaven knows what—what is wrong? *I have now started to see an occasional movie.* I now have no nightmares, and life for me is wonderful. It seems so strange—a prayer, then meeting you, *and getting medicine that has changed my life so much!*

11-1-57   Sunday I start work—this time *as a waitress, in an institution.* And my nurse friends, as usual, are horrified. In all this period of resting, I prayed that *as long as I live I would be granted the privilege of being of service to others.* I am deeply, sincerely thankful that God showed me this— either walk out or collapse mentally. And what means the most in my life is to know you and your secretaries and to be cared for by you. My mind is healed; my ears no more hear the screaming of helpless children who cannot talk, with the heartbreaking look in their eyes.

No wonder poor women again and again have babies—it's the only time they get cared for as a person.

Pride in one's work is good. *I like people,* and when one can walk out of hell with a mind still able to rest, to laugh and live again—fine.

11-2-57 And I have the riches of two good feet with plenty of lovely places to walk to; and I can laugh again; and I have nerves that are calmed down, and I have courage. I AM NOT WASTING TIME ON BEING UNHAPPY, because I don't see anything I can't give up. I have fought a battle with my nerves, to develop the deep resources within myself, and not hurt my family. I like to be attractive. My attacks of depression still come, but who doesn't have them?

This morning, after being up for a while, *I had a very severe attack of dizziness. The table got to whirling slowly, but I was wise; I sat on the floor. If I die I want to be alone.* None of this excitement and being given stimulants. In a way *I died too long ago really to care now about things that are nothing to me.* But I'll never let you down. *I pray only that I go out of this world before I end up senile, a body but no mind.*

This is the first time in my life that I am thinking clearly, facing facts; and I can laugh.

11-6-57 Now comes the story of all my adventures. I never knew that I could raise hell and be so mean. Well, I arrived in my new place to work for this family, and I had a fight with the damned fool woman who didn't know that I was to live in her house. But her remarks, her manners—so I said, "Fine; I just came from the city, and it's just as easy to go back." And I looked full of hell, too. She calmed down. First day at work I was stared at.

I look at myself, an alive, glowing woman; I look at the nurses I wait on—exhausted or damned fat and sloppy. I enjoy seeing what looks like me in the mirror. You took the veil from my eyes and set me free to live and breathe. *Life is an adventure; I mean to get all I can out of it. The hell with the good woman bunk.*

11-8-57   I realize this: I can't have everything my way in this world—and I can't run around quitting jobs.

Today I took a good look at what I have learned so far. The cheap wages, the exploited people. Women so lazy— who refuse to accept being responsible for their husband and children. But out of all this, I have made one definite decision—never, as long as I live, will a penny of mine go to charity. I am not bitter—but I have had a good look at frightened people, who huddle so close together—with fear showing in the way they speak and act. And all they can boast of is, "My husband and I are college graduates." When I sat in a state agency, looking for domestic work, when I saw what is accepted into their homes so Mrs. Snob can gossip with her friends—I have had it.

And always these words—you must work faster. I didn't say anything, but in the afternoon when I finally sat down for a few minutes I was worn out. But I was quiet: I never argued; I just studied the setup and told myself, to hell with this town.

And *on duty I started to have tremors in both arms.* Off duty *slight convulsive feelings,* but my mind—picture after picture of strange, fantastic colors, birds, flowers. *Last night my whole face started to jerk; usually I start with a little twitching about the mouth.* [INTERESTING THAT MUCH FATIGUE BROUGHT BACK SOME OF RUTH'S OLD EPILEPTIC TROUBLES.]

11-9-57   I am fine—I just let that woman in charge fuss, and to be very honest, I didn't hear a damned word.

My arms are still jerking as I write—some slight tremors. I think a lot of this is due to poor food. But I never believe in arguments. With the mentality of these people, why waste time? I have honestly enjoyed my week here. It was work, but stimulating and healthy. But when I developed tremors in my arms in the daytime, and slight convulsions started, it was best to get out quick. I did not know this school was for the helpless—with no minds. God forgot to finish their faces. *I can't take that. I can't stand looking at these helpless people. What I can do quickly, they do slowly.* Must my life be spent in a world of problems? I prefer to look at real, everyday people. But the people here, I can truthfully say, have been very nice to me. But I'll keep looking for another place.

For two nights I have had this experience. I could hear in my mind many voices talking, laughing, screaming. Last night, as the pictures began to form and change, I wanted to scream and run. But I am careful; I take the medicine as you told me to. I will admit that inside my mind, I was burned up.

Well, I have no regrets—I do admire myself for this ability to make a decision—act and go, and not brood. What is over with is just another experience. And I did no talking —I just kept quiet. But I am not a person that any damned woman can *destroy mentally*. When it gets rough I do this: again I look back to the first time I came, so frightened, to you. Cancer was the least of my troubles—but dear God— my MIND! Did I have any? Well, I have honestly, truthfully enjoyed my week here. *I think it showed one thing—my new lack of fear in facing life.*

11-12-57   Today I went for an interview. The dog took one look at me, stood up and tried to give me a kiss and then crawled into my lap. The wife told me I would get room and board and occasionally have to care for the children.

Last night about 8 P.M. tremors began in my arms, and my body felt ready to take off. I took more Dilantin and got out of the house quick. When I came back in a few minutes I was fine. The storms in my mind are getting quieter.

I did raise 19 kinds of hell about living conditions in the last place where I stayed. I guess I didn't do myself much good. *I cried a lot, but what good will that do?*

Dr. Alvarez, should I run far and hide? There was a woman, a waitress, with the most pitiful heartbroken look on her face—so lost, so alone. I didn't talk to her. But you know me—I study people's faces; I did not know she was pregnant. But then I learned that she was. I wrote to her, told her she could get help and would not have to pay. I tried to write as I would have written to stand by a daughter. Is it wrong to feel that perhaps God wanted me to help this poor girl?

I have known terror when no matter how kind the doctor, receptionist, nurse, was, all I wanted to do was get out faster than I came in.

If only somewhere I could hold a lovely child in my arms, and look at nomal children.

11-12-57   But what a relief—medicine to calm my mind so I can listen and understand what you say—to be guided and shown where my danger lies. *But this is what means the most to me—not to be afraid.*

11-13-57   I sent forth my brothers as men into the world, not sniveling brats that could not take life. If I had sons, they would learn to stand up and face life. If any woman makes unpleasant remarks to me, I leave a bitter curse behind when I leave, that she will eat in bitterness and have tears in her bread. Now I am going to see to it that there are no children where I work; I have had enough of them.

11-27-57   THANKSGIVING DAY.

This is the problem I have had, and it's easing quite a bit. I did begin to get nervous in the house alone, but I decided since the dog was quiet there was nothing to be afraid of. But I have been having some slight stormy mental tensions; it's as if two minds struggle for mastery. *And I get the feeling of wanting to harm someone, but this does not come up as strongly as that which I faced in the past. When I was at home alone, visiting with my niece, I looked at the kitchen knife and I thought, "Why not make an end for two?"* I realize that I have these storms in my mind, but *I feel I can control myself.* The heartbreaking battle before I came to you was terrifying to me. But I do avoid newspaper articles about murder, where people say they couldn't control their impulses. When I read them I feel frightened. [A NUMBER OF EPILEPTICS HAVE TOLD OF THESE IMPULSES THAT CAME TO THEM TO KILL SOMEONE.]

Last night it seemed to me as I lay in bed that I could hear a storm of voices, and I wanted to scream. Last night I saw an array of horrors as I started falling asleep. My trouble was that I failed to take my night dose of Dilantin by falling asleep. The result was that I woke with a bad dream; also I got a headache.

11-28-57 I won't write much today because I have found out that housework is not easy. I am in a home with wonderful people. I can be myself—relaxed, quiet and calm. I like it here. It's such a pretty home. And it's wonderful to live with a family where everybody talks quietly and with courtesy. I am getting adjusted to the job—being a waitress for the week before helped me. I am satisfied. The doctor's wife cooks such lovely food. Strange, but I feel all the old way of life of my childhood. I am treated with courtesy. The doctor walks in—and he gives me the newspaper. This may not seem like much but to me it's wonderful—*I am accepted.*

11-29-57 I am fine—I am letting myself relax, to absorb the beauty and quiet of my new life. There are two children—a girl 5 years, a boy 10. I am amazed that children can be so nice. I feel as if I had lived here all my life. The doctor's wife said I could call her by her first name, but I said I would prefer that we kept it on a Mrs. and Ruth basis. We don't talk a lot—there is a quiet courtesy between us, and it's wonderful. Well, I had a good year of mental discipline. And in this home I will learn to be a good housekeeper.

You, Doctor, have done so much for me, I no longer feel shy, I feel just calm and quiet.

12-5-57   I do get restless, and occasionally feel trapped; but I get a breath of fresh air as I open the kitchen window, and I can always go out of doors. I am beginning to feel young again, and not as stiff; I seldom have a backache.

I could never, however, without my medicine, have made the grade. When I am too long without it, I notice it. I hear in my mind my name called out loud—many voices speak. But I don't worry. The most wonderful gain to me last night was my lack of fear in being out alone in the dark. As usual, I didn't check directions too closely, but I knew how to get back; the sense of panic was not present.

My ears and face occasionally burn as if I am being roasted; I guess it's hot flushes.

12-6-57   I shall get more out of life than a warm smile and lovely hair. And if I don't dream of how to enjoy being alive, think what might happen; I might lose an opportunity to meet that man with $56 million. I have heard that there are two millionaires in this town—each one of them owns a bank. It may be wise to open a small account in each bank. I think I will. Am I a designing hussy? Well, this is my chance to learn how to run a home.

12-9-57   I am getting along well and I am happy in this work. The sudden jumpy movements of my arms, dropping things, are now rarely coming. I am learning to cook.

I wake up each morning with numbness in my hands. And I had a mental vision of two deep blue serious eyes gazing at me. I just kept quiet, and went ahead preparing dinner. I must have good nerves; I just acted as usual—quiet, friendly, relaxed.

12-24-57 I am getting better adjusted mentally and physically. Christmas tomorrow—and it's certainly exciting in this place. I am getting along, and my right arm is fine. I just have never paid attention to numbness; but the sense of touch is so weak, that picking up things is not easy. And there are problems with speech; periods of blankness. But all is now easing up. Without my Dilantin I would never have come this far. I have an idea from occasional dizzy attacks and the feeling that a weight rests on my head, that my blood pressure has taken its often upward swing. I don't worry about it, just a problem to live with, and I can be happy as a lark. *The feeling in my right arm is coming back.*

12-30-57 When I first started here I dropped and broke everything. *My speech was bad—I couldn't talk properly.* I had much mental confusion. Words not pronounced right; blankness; sentences formed and repeated over and over. But I knew I could and would make the grade. I took the little girl here and a neighbor's son out. We went to the park, so the children could go sledding. *Who fell six times? Me, of course, in my best coat.* Walking across the lawn, down I went. The dog ran up to see if I was *O.K.*

Chapter III—1958

1-8-58   One day I forgot to take my medicine, and hallucinations began. I saw a strange face, like a monster of some kind, bloated and smiling above a cupboard. At times I feel like crying and saying, "What's the use?" But I remember your words, "Life is a battle and must be fought each day."

A friend says I am a dreamer. I agree, but the dreamy moments are simply the times when I am suddenly "not around." [THIS IS A DESCRIPTION OF PETIT MAL.] I would like to fly again in a plane, high above the clouds. Regardless of whether there is a heaven or hell, why should I sit and mourn and prepare for my grave or cremation? I hate gossip, and the bitterness and meanness of some people. Should I be thankful? For what? Getting older, finding myself stiffer and stiffer, and out of breath when I walk?

And how happy I would be to get myself a new brain that is good. Writing to you is giving me a chance to work off the tension, and also the self-pity. I am just letting myself go and showing you my conflicts and my worries. I work hard, but that is good for me; I need to. Again I have a family, people who understand me. Too long did I live alone, hiding from the world. It was foolish. Now I face a challenge and I won't let you down.

I still have this problem: I am slowed up mentally. I couldn't stand radio music or the children's programs on television until I took my medicine.

Suppose I leave. Where would I go? And for what? I'll be damned if I'll sit back and worry. The time to laugh, to live, is now. How soon will I be dead? I am saving for a trip, because someday it will be my last. I never wanted to live or come back to life. Well, I am here, but for what? To look at the hell people love? To support innocent, helpless children? Books, music, I have no time for that.

1-13-58   I am so damned tired of acting as if nothing ever hurt me. Don't worry; I'll never harm anyone.

2-1-58   At long last I can let go and cry, but the problem is this: suddenly on the street, in the house, tears fall like a gentle rain. Once I let a child steal my heart, and I promised myself, Never again. My mind at long last must have a rest. I have given until I can't give any more.

I go so quickly from one mood to another, I amaze myself. But the physical work is the best thing that ever happened to me.

I get worried, frightened—about what, I don't know. I get ready to leave, run, and go. Then I tell myself that the door is now closed. Let's stand up and be a success instead of a frightened child. [MANY AN EPILEPTIC SPEAKS OF THESE SUDDEN FEARS OF HE KNOWS NOT WHAT.]

Once in a while I see two of every single object. I am sleeping well since I decided to be a nudist again. I hate clothes at night.

2-19-58   I fell the other day and hurt both hands, and I was madder than hell. Life to me is "Watch out! Watch out!" The other day as I turned off the electric range, my left hand jumped, and I burned two fingers. I am going through a period of not being able to hold anything. It seems that my hands just let go. But now I have a new talent; as an object drops from the left hand, I catch it with the right hand.

2-24-58   I have made up my mind, no more trying to go without my medicine. When I cut down on it, I am mentally lost. [MANY PATIENTS GET INTO TROUBLE BY ALWAYS TRYING TO CUT DOWN ON THE AMOUNT OF MUCH-NEEDED MEDICINE THEY TAKE. RUTH WOULD HAVE BEEN MUCH BETTER

OFF IF REGULARLY, EVERY DAY, SHE HAD TAKEN THE FOUR DILANTIN CAPSULES I HAD PRESCRIBED. BUT SHE SAID SHE DIDNT WANT TO "GET DEPENDENT" ON THE MEDICINE.]

I had a dream in which I wanted so much to hold a child, and a little one came into my arms. The warmth, the love; and beside him stood one of my former precious darlings. His eyes were so sad, the little face was so wistful. I woke up before I could talk to him and tell him what it meant to me to meet him again.

Hell, I get sick of life—trying and trying. The other day I was so angry at Walter Winchell and his broadcast that I lit two burners and just missed burning a wooden handle on a pot. This is one time anger was my trouble.

3-5-58   I must have beauty in my life. Since you took my hand and showed me, I can go unafraid. I still have the hellish attacks of temper. My employers say too damned many "Do this's" and "Do that's."

I realize that I am a problem to myself, to you and Dr. Hyman, but since when is it wrong to be me and no one else?

3-6-58   I feel trapped and frightened when my hands jump. I fall or stumble, or kick a rug. This damned house— I am leaving; I can't take it any more. For what? Why argue or fuss? I'll get dressed and go.

3-7-58   I seem to have awakened from a deep shock. At long last I have less tremor and am able to put things down without breaking them. One day I even put the little girl's shirts in the refrigerator. Always I must be on guard; I become so confused. I apologized to my boss, and told him I was afraid I was mentally ill.

3-9-58   My decision is made: I will QUIT as soon as my boss and his wife are home. Suddenly my brain feels flamingly alive—as I have never been in all my life. My fear of facing life is gone. I feel wonderful. One day, I seemed to have wakened from a trance. The falling and dizziness have cleared up.

3-11-58 I just talked to the nicest policeman I ever met. That lovely bit of an Irish brogue—I was enchanted. Well, we exchanged views and thoughts. I am really practicing; perhaps I'll find myself in the lovely modern kitchen of a millionaire. I still like housework; I am not cured of that. Nursing for me is out, and I have no regrets; I nursed for 31 years, and that's enough. I am going to take it easy for one month; it seems to me at long last I know the meaning of life—its ups and downs.

All my life I have wanted to have some place in which I could just relax and enjoy nature, away from people. Often I have been terrified of being out of work. I don't know where I got the idea I have to save and save. Once a waiter told me, "One half of your life is gone; the second each day brings closer to an end. So live and enjoy yourself now." And I do. I have two dear friends, each one married, worried, upset, afraid to spend or laugh. I have time to read the newspaper, to get books at the library. I am enjoying myself. Today I have no place to go except to look at the lake later in the day. God in his time will place me where I should be. Slavery is out. And mentally my brain is quiet. Because a man is master (or thinks he is), mentally he makes women slaves. I feel unafraid when I can ask questions and meet people. This is the way I brought up my youngest brother, who didn't talk until he was four.

3-14-58 I am starting to write letters to my friends. My letters are written much better. When I write to you, it's getting out all the built-up tension, the fear, anger, and so forth. I feel wonderful; I did not realize how starved I was for books, companionship and sleep.

When I am calm I write small, neatly; but when I get

excited, boiling mad, the words run so fast in my mind I can't put them down well. Who has time then for spelling?

3-20-58   I will never forget the time I was on the main street of a small town, and two little boys—monsters—tried to throw me down. I wanted then to throw them down on the pavement.

3-21-58   The manager of this hotel is keeping her eye on me. Once that would have had me moving out damned quick; I just never could stand the thought that anyone dared to think I could not walk alone. But her warm kisses, hugs, coffee, cookies, a chance to talk, and now it's not wrong to accept kindness, at long last.

3-22-58   I have not been just tired—I was frightened, exhausted, and damned fed up. To live with a woman who does not realize that marriage today should be more than slavery—hell! You can keep it. I am willing to work, but I'll be damned if any slaving wife will drag me down.

3-26-58   This morning I wakened—no headache, and my hands are getting steady. *I realize the honor you do me in wanting me to have an autobiographical book.*

3-27-58   This is the first time in my life that I am getting acquainted with myself as a woman who is free from fear, and I am learning the value of rest as I have never known it.

4-4-58   In this great city a certain man and his son do not know it, but I am going to be just the woman they need to make a home for them. I have found I can't retire into a shell; I am afraid of taking money out of the bank to live on. My winter of work taught me much.

As far as sex is concerned, I know nothing. My new employer: if he feels that I could be kissed occasionally, fine. Go ahead. That means nothing to me. A man from the church offered to set me up in a little apartment and said he would take care of me. I just had no feeling about it. Alone,

I'll be able to plan my own work, and that for me is very important. And then there will be no one to be shocked when I sleep nude. A towel covering a woman when she is not overweight still makes her a lot more eye-catching than a woman with nothing on.

4-9-58 I found that as soon as I cut down on the dosage of Dilantin, I began to go right back to worrying, to wanting to walk out of doors at night.

4-10-58 Because I left off taking my medicine I had to spend a day in bed; I could not stand or walk. My head was going into space; my mind was saying, "Lie down." So I did. I just lay on the floor. I decided that if I was going to die, then I preferred to be alone.

Later, I took a good look in the mirror to see why I had been letting my head fall to the side after all the falls and pain I had had. I had never noticed, but the mirror showed the right shoulder lower than the left. I said to myself, "I am going to make my shoulder be straight." Fine; walk. And then the head went on the side again. I know that any woman who is afraid to say, "Is there something wrong?" has never grown up.

4-11-58 My jaws snapped; I just feel the inside of my mouth twitching, and somehow I kept from biting my tongue. Now I am all right again.

4-16-58 Suddenly I hear a voice in my mind; over and over it calls "Ruth." Because of the long-ago night when my brother called me in an hour of danger, I prayed. Afterwards he told me that he heard my voice and fear left him. People today think prayer is a joke. I never found it so.

My father and I were two unhappy people when together. We were both hot-tempered, stubborn, impossible to live with each other. The day came when he left me and never came back. But as the years passed, my classmate suggested that I find my father and make friends. For that I shall always be grateful to her. When I saw the condition my father lived in, I decided it was his life, not mine. We each had the right to go our own way.

This is the first time in my life I have been lazy and have stayed in bed until 11 A.M. or 12 noon, and it doesn't worry me.

Whenever I meet hungry people, I'll help them; I have to live calmly, I know, but I just got fed up with it.

4-20-58 I found when I lessen the dose of Dilantin the tremors I have are the beginning of trouble. Often when I sit to read a book, I keep reaching out for a fly that isn't there.

Now I must face the truth. I cannot walk without falling. For me this is a new road—where it goes I don't know. But I will not go to work where I can endanger the lives of helpless people.

You may ask yourself if it was worthwhile to have accepted me as a patient. What are my thoughts? Two wonderful years of sleep without nightmares. To be able to make decisions, from buying a pair of shoes to taking a vacation. Trying to walk to the bathroom is like a journey to far-off places.

My family have asked me to come over, but I can't. They would get upset, and for what? I have always stood alone; I have been proud. I am thinking, Why not go to the United Charities Association? They have trained social workers. I must plan to live where I can earn and not be a burden. I am thankful for the most beautiful words a doctor can speak, your words, "I can help you."

It is wonderful—no longer to swear. I thank the good God for the hour he sent me to you, and that I alone in my family face this problem. You have always told me the truth. Never have you spoken lightly; and it's up to me. I realize that no one helps himself by wanting to die, but I am bitter and fed up.

I have thought and asked myself time and again, shall I just drop out of sight once and for all? But where does one go? What good will it do? My ears are ringing.

Somewhere in my brain is this strange feeling I once had—a darkness that I would never emerge from. There is only one thing—it's too bad man has not invented what is needed most—a button to press, and that will be the end.

4-21-58 [THIS REMARKABLE DOCUMENT OF A PERSON WHO THOUGHT SHE WAS DYING—FOUND AFTER HER DEATH IN HER SAFETY DEPOSIT BOX. THIS TIME RUTH WAS WRONG; SHE STILL HAD SEVERAL YEARS IN WHICH TO LIVE.] Forgive me; I must talk to my brothers, and in memory again we are five frightened children. Then and now all I have to say is this: do not feel sorry or shed tears. I am deeply happy; my hour has come to go home. My doctors—so wise and dear.

Dear Brother E. Your precious little daughter I shall not be around to meet, but I love her dearly. My new sister—kiss her most tenderly and tell her this: I am sorry. God called me home. It is best so for me. I have walked a long road; my feet are weary. Now the time has come for eternal rest. But I have known love so deep and sincere, part of God's great plan to help others. I have no sorrow. What woman can have the joy I have had? When morning comes I shall have gone home. I have prayed for this hour, and to me it has been granted. I am to be cremated, as my will states. My ashes scattered. And the dearest and greatest of doctors—to be remembered—he has done so much for me. Comfort my brothers A. and E. Each one of you, love Brother A. for the person he is. But there are to be no tears. I am tired.

Do this for me; there are two lovely women in Dr. Alvarez's office. To Estelle please give my butterflies and the little wristwatch to Dorothy, and the other sweet woman working there must have my little totem pole.

In the event I am found dead, please notify my doctors. They may wish to do an autopsy to find out what my brain shows. They know, I know, that I am progressing more rapidly into whatever is wrong; I go without fear. I have known for a long time I will die; there is no fear, no sadness. I am not dying from a broken heart because I left the children at the clinic.

It's night—3:30 A.M. April 21, 1958. In my top drawers I leave two letters. I was too tired to write more. But my dear and wonderful Dr. Alvarez—may the dear God bless and keep him safe. He gave me two of the loveliest years. Under his care I have been able to work. In this hotel, anyone whose feelings I have hurt, please forgive me. I came back to die. That I have known.

Publish in the *Tribune* that I am dead . . . all my clothes will go to the Salvation Army.

Don't be sorry; I am glad to die. This headache is the beginning of what is to be the end.

These people—let them know I am dead. [THEN FOLLOWS A LIST OF HER FRIENDS.] I go home to God with love for all of you. My headache is returning strangely. But I shall go to sleep. I have had happiness beyond price. All of you I love dearly, but I will go back to bed. Blurred are my eyes. The words swim and I see them, then I don't. When I pass through this lovely golden light, never to come back, I am cared for. For me you made it a world of laughter. You showed me that I had a mind with which to think. I am tired, I fought sincerely to go on, but now the time has come to go home. I have known for a long time my road was death. I have had the greatest joy—babies in my arms, children to call me "Mamma." Aged people to say a rosary for me.

Yes, this I know—in this hour when one accepts the way

of the cross, *you* know, if there is anything in this book that will help many others to go on, then I have given something, and I can go home in gladness and joy. My life—it is over.

4-26-58 I had an attack of high blood pressure and was in the hospital a short time. Today my family came to me; I agreed to go home and run the house while my brother had surgery for his hernia. But then I began to feel depressed. I can't stand living in my brother's house. He fusses over me. My sister-in-law is lovely, but we have a slight personality clash. [A MOST UNUSUAL AND REMARKABLE THING ABOUT RUTH WAS THAT TIME AND AGAIN SHE THOUGHT OF GETTING A LAWYER TO ASK A COURT TO TELL HER BROTHERS TO QUIT TRYING TO TAKE GOOD CARE OF HER!!] How does one divorce a brother who doesn't seem to understand that nobody asked him to do anything? All the other members of my family, we just live our lives. Friday I leave—I have had enough. Up to now I have been courteous. But if necessary, a lawyer may settle our problem. My brother and his wife insist I stay with them. But, Dr. Alvarez, at my age, does one have to get a lawyer to get one's family out of one's life? [CURIOUSLY, RUTH AT TIMES SEEMED PARANOIAC, THINKING HER BROTHER, WHEN HE KEPT TRYING TO HELP HER, WAS ANNOYING HER SO MUCH SHE WOULD NEED LEGAL PROTECTION! IT SHOWS HOW TRE-MENDOUSLY INDEPENDENT SHE ALWAYS WAS. AS SHE SAID ONCE, IF SHE WERE MARRIED AND HER HUSBAND WERE TO ASK, "WHERE WERE YOU THIS AFTERNOON?" SHE WOULD WALK RIGHT OUT ON HIM.]

4-27-58 This period of stormy emotion brought pain such as I haven't known since you started to care for me. I got up to take medicine, and to get across the floor was not easy. The back of my ears began to throb.

I am deeply sorry, Dr. Alvarez, what lies ahead I don't know; but please accept my grateful thanks. I pray and ask God—let me die now while I can walk, and yet, who am I to dare to ask? If I am to go, now has begun my real battle.

This type of headache I have not had since you started to care for me. Please do not fear that I took more medicine than I should have.

4-28-58   It's strange to me; each time I am supposed to make a change, I get ill.

4-30-58   I never worry; I find it wise not to walk down steps without holding onto a banister. I can easily walk up steps.

5-3-58   I am at my brother's home. I feel I am not breathing. My heart suddenly starts to beat hard; to walk is not easy. I received a pretty bad blow. Last evening at home I was looking into a mirror and as I freshened up, my face was so distorted in appearance, so long and gray. Then I started to fall, but I caught myself.

I am extremely restless at night. I frankly have no desire to fight any more. I feel like a person that is standing watching someone else struggling. Again tonight, my feet burn.

5-10-58   It's nice out here at my brother's home. But each day brings a headache so bad I can't move my head. Strange, I was putting up a battle, but my mind was disappearing. Now again I feel like a quiet woman. I get along well with the family. I just keep quiet. I try to live in the world of people, but this is one change I have not been able to accept; I must be me, the person I am, but my family goes their way, I go mine. It is best so.

5-25-58   [RUTH SEEMS TO HAVE HAD SOME MORE SMALL STROKES. APPARENTLY SHE FOUND A NEW PLACE TO WORK IN.] At 1 P.M. I began to have a very severe pain in my right foot. My foot wants to draw up as I try to walk; pain goes up to back of the knee, along the leg. I am waking with numbness in my hands. In trying to pick up anything, occasionally I get severe pain. Right hand is very hard to cope with, very weak and numb.

I like my new home. It's a lot of work, but I don't mind that. With a lot of electrical gadgets, I am not overworked. It's just this awful pain that I can't ignore; I *have* it.

6-1-58 Three mornings ago I fell against the bathtub. All I have to do is walk around and I get hurt. *My body jumps so suddenly* I am thrown off my feet and don't know what happens. [OFTEN I HAVE DIAGNOSED EPILEPSY FROM THIS STORY.]

6-3-58 I awoke about 3 A.M. Monday to realize I was coming out of a bad seizure of some sort. I was lying on my back, my arms and legs were wildly jumping in the air. Bedclothes were on the floor. The last thing I remembered was a slight twitching around my lips, and I thought, Be careful. This may be a convulsion. I finally woke up enough to find my arms and legs calming down, and I was on the bed. Hungry—I was starved, restless, wide awake. I wanted to go out at 3 A.M. and walk real fast, any place—just to go. I got up with care; I could walk, so I made a cup of Sanka, then went back to sleep. It's hell I fight, knowing that I can fall suddenly, have a convulsion. I am lucky—my family never saw me in a seizure.

6-6-58 [AS I HAVE SAID BEFORE, RUTH SOMETIMES STOPPED TAKING HER MEDICINE AND THEN USUALLY PAID IN MUCH SUFFERING FOR THIS. SHE STOPPED HER MEDICINE THIS TIME SO THAT HER FAMILY WOULD NOT KEEP ASKING, "WHAT ARE YOU TAKING AND WHY?"] I never told Dr. Hyman I was off Dilantin for the past two months. All I wanted was never to see my family again, and to get away. I am not an easy person for any doctor to care for.

Since having this difficult spell, I feel quiet and relaxed.

I'll go along for a while, then suddenly something happens to my brain. I get into trouble because I get confused. I feel like a fool. It's hard for me to ever admit that I am not well.

7-12-58   I quit this job today. I'll never on earth satisfy this woman. Yesterday I became quite dizzy and fell down on the street. I couldn't even get up. Two men came to my aid; a policeman was called and he took me to a doctor. I feel a lot of my problems are from being overtired. When I went back on Dilantin I had a severe reaction; my mouth became very sore.

I hope I never see this woman again. I feel fine this morning since I decided to leave. I cannot live in mental torture any longer.

7-14-58   I have thought about going back to nursing but *I hate it*. I am going to learn to be a good housemaid. I don't mind the work; physically I am healthy, but I have to work out my mental attitude.

Today my vision is blurred; I saw two of everything. I don't give a damn. Last week a bus nearly got me.

The homes of my brothers are now open to me, and I'll never say any but nice things about my sisters-in-law. As long as my family knows nothing of my illness, I'll be O.K. My brother gets upset, sheds tears, and then fights with me. My job is giving me a nice inferiority complex. Just thinking of being back in uniform makes me feel better.

7-22-58   This morning I got into a mean mood before I became dizzy. I felt like writing my brother a nasty letter. But I remember what you said, "Write the letter, then tear it up."

7-24-58   I am so glad that I never fell that time with the six-month-old baby in my arms. That almost happened one morning. After that I lived in fear each time I picked him up.

Here are the problems I got into; one morning after I

had breakfast my arm suddenly jumped, my hand hit a plate and knocked it on the floor. The dishes belong to a set and can't be replaced. I felt sick even though these people were nice about it. At night I cried, I was so lonely. I was just the maid, someone to work, and that is all.

Well, I am slowed down now; my mind feels alert, and I promise I'll never again fight or argue. I do have hell's own temper. As time goes on, I see the type of brain I must live with, and then I try to be wiser.

7-28-58   Ambition is coming back; I feel like working. I am stubborn; I should not be a maid.

8-6-58   No snob I work for will ever again walk over my heart. I believe in being a good Christian but that does not mean, turn the other cheek. No one at any time will slap my cheek.

8-10-58   It seems I am always trying to break my bones or commit suicide. I fell on a pavement; my heel slipped, and down I went. I was so disgusted I cried, but since you have cured me of swearing, I just had no words to say! I have had a year of falls.

8-21-58   Today my mind went blank in public. I tried to ask the waitress for a cup of coffee. Twice all I could say was "Hot." I felt strange; my mind was just a blank. She was kind and started to try and help me get straightened out. But I managed to say, "Black coffee." The lady sitting near me, the waitress, and I, laughed. I said something about my sitting daydreaming. It's the only way I can ever cover up. I just pretend that this is nothing out of the ordinary. But too well do I know the truth. Since I have been resting, I have had no trouble mentally. Today was the first time in ages I had such an attack. And as usual, I have now gone to another domestic agency to get a new job.

8-22-58   I am going back to nursing—a stronger woman mentally and physically.

8-24-58   After two days of thinking, I knew that nursing and I are finished. I still prefer to scrub a floor instead of giving a patient a bath.

9-3-58 [FOUND IN RUTH'S SAFETY DEPOSIT BOX AFTER SHE DIED.] What are the words one can say —thank you for your kindness and understanding; and courtesy in not probing too deeply into questions and problems. [A PHYSICIAN MUST BE ABLE TO SENSE WHEN HE HAD BETTER STOP ASKING QUESTIONS.] I realized I walked deeply into the forest of a darkness that now I run from. So much I should once have known—now too late comes the knowledge; and to me is life worth living? Frankly, no. For what? The scales have fallen long since from my eyes. Lord, let me go now. Yes, that is selfish. But what does one get for being unselfish? I am too tired to be bitter, and all I pray is, Lord, may I go to sleep and never waken. I am sick of looking back. I am now finished.

9-13-58 I think this is the first time in my life I just stopped running and sat down. Since I can now walk properly, I behave, and especially I take my medicine.

10-8-58 I visited every employment agency, but decided nursing is out.

I can often see the difference that Dilantin and Mebaral make in me. [OFTEN I THINK HOW STRANGE IT IS THAT MANY PATIENTS KEEP STOPPING THE TAKING OF THEIR MEDICINE LONG AFTER THEY HAVE SEEN THAT THEY WILL PAY HEAVILY FOR THAT.]

[HERE IS SOMETHING THAT RUTH RARELY EVER SAID.] Now I want a life like other women; to really make myself attractive, cut my hair, and get married. I have had enough of being alone. Taking care of a husband is better than discussing a book with oneself.

10-11-58 I had an interview for a job caring for a patient who has high blood pressure and hardening of the arteries. But a small town makes me feel I am fenced in. Caring for someone, however, is fine.

Salespeople get annoyed at me. I have trouble with speech. I don't know what I was going to ask for. I ask for directions, and then I can't at times understand them. [OFTEN RUTH WOULD CROSS A STREET AGAINST A LIGHT.] One morning I went out for a paper. Lights were changing for me to walk. I never read a paper as I cross, so I can't figure this out: I was halfway on the pavement, reading the paper. I felt myself come back, and I said, "What goes on?" I don't worry about these problems. I can more often now catch myself in time.

10-19-58　　About 3 or 4 months ago I met a nurse's aid, Rose, a nice woman, and I had lunch with her. When I got sick, she came to visit me, and brought me flowers. Fear slightly began to enter my mind. She called me and her voice had a possessive tone on the phone. She loaned me gowns, a robe, we wrote notes.

One day Rose cried and told me she had no money and was hungry. I insisted she come in with me. One thing I noticed; we gave each other a kiss and a hug as if we hadn't seen each other for a long time. I was relaxed; she held herself so stiff, and cool. Later, when I came home, Rose said, "You are pretty." I can't say that is an unusual remark; I have said that to women I meet, but . . . one time she had said, "You will never have to worry about money."

One time, as she sat across the room from me, her light-blue eyes became a murky, dirty gray. My thoughts: Does she plan to knife or shoot me? So I got up and insisted Rose must have a cup of coffee with me. And as she stood in the doorway, I felt guilty to think that I thought of her as wanting to harm me. I had an impulse to kiss her goodnight. But that kind of impulse I never fool with. I know that there are times that I, as an unmarried woman, have feelings one doesn't proclaim. And I don't plan to take on the nearest man to take on my emotions.

This was the last night I saw Rose. Next night, I am told, she knocked at my door, but I did not let her in; I was dead asleep. Next day I got home at 7 P.M. Rose was found in her room dead, eyes closed, bedclothes covering her neatly. Can it be possible that she was a lesbian? Who am I to say? I can say to you honestly and sincerely I did nothing wrong.

Rose had begun to like the taste of liquor; I sensed that she had been in love with some girl. I saw enough of lesbians in training. Only once did a girl get too affectionate with me, and I threw her on the floor. [RUTH AT TIMES FORGOT THAT ONCE WHEN ANOTHER LESBIAN NURSE MADE ADVANCES, RUTH REPORTED HER TO HER SUPERIOR.]

10-20-58   This worries me—the lawyer Rose had in the city knew her sad history, and discussed it with me. I hope the newspapers do not get the story. Before God I say that we were just two lonely women, trying to help each other. She told her lawyer often how happy she had been when with me. As far as I am concerned, I have nothing to regret; I am glad that for a little while a lonely woman found laughter and kindness. It is a mystery to me how Rose came to die. She had her bedclothes neatly arranged over her.

10-25-58   [AT TIMES RUTH'S WRITING SHOW-ED HER MENTAL CONFUSION.] I sincerely appecil (can't spell—feel confused; it's like a blank or as if a light went off. I know how to spell these simple words, but my brain can't tell my hand to write correctly.) Today I have not been able to tell time, but I don't worry; my brain is in a confused state. I realize my greatest need now is for people.

Last night Mrs. W. and I had a talk. I went to bed so restless I forgot to take my medicine; I took it at 11 P.M., but half an hour later I was so restless I took more. I was lying on my face, thinking. Then I got this sudden crash, like a tornado, or how can I say it? I was not asleep, just in the darkness. Then two children appeared—small, but they looked so old; their faces were drawn. I heard myself moan out loud; I felt jerking from my neck down. Then the grimacing and making faces stopped. Then once again clouds, so strange and pretty, came—black with lines of white. Dancers appeared—beautiful young girls in bird costumes. Their bodies and faces were going through contortions.

10-29-58   Yesterday I moved from the hotel to a small apartment. The minute I came through the door I knew I was ready to leave forever. There is something in this room that is strange. It's just like the time I felt someone was in my apartment, and then later on, I felt a warm hand clasp mine. I then did what any good mid-Victorian maiden would have done; I fainted. I have no fear, except I feel now and then that something is strange around me; but then again, it's gone.

11-11-58   My mind is coming to life. My greatest desire now is to take dancing lessons. I love music; I love to see people dance. Well, one of these days I'll get disgusted; I shall do as a shy woman did; pay for lessons all at one time. I must learn to dance.

12-16-58   Six days ago I visited with my family. We were very happy. They brought me home.

12-23-58   You brought me out of a world of fear, Dr. Alvarez, and I don't plan to go back into it. I refuse to die by my own hand. Yes, I do have periods of suddenly having just a blank mind.

12-25-58   Before the school fire [THERE WAS A TERRIBLE FIRE IN A PAROCHIAL SCHOOL WHERE MANY CHILDREN WERE KILLED.], I felt at times that something terrible or bad would happen. I couldn't shake off this feeling. After the school tragedy I was finally O.K., but the shock! I couldn't watch television or read; all I did was cry.

Chapter IV—1959

1-11-59　　On going to bed, suddenly, a ghastly, immense man with one blue eye—a cyclops—appeared. Dark clouds, voices, talking continuously, faces, I felt a deep shudder, then deep into sleep until morning.

1-16-59　　I now, after going to housekeeping, am a different woman. Scrubbing a floor seems better than caring for the sick.

2-20-59　　I listen to religious services on the radio. They terrify me, because I can't help it; I want to argue right back. No religion should be pushed down one's throat.

2-23-59　　I went home and had a wonderful visit with my family.

4-10-59　　Last night the maid told me that a man, in a rage, had struck his wife. I felt sick. The day a man strikes me I'll kill him, if it's the last thing I live to do.

In this world, there will never be enough room for two women in one household. [THE CHINESE CHARACTER, OR WRITING SIGN, FOR "TROUBLE" IS TWO WOMEN UNDER ONE ROOF.]

4-11-59　　I have no man's shoulder to cry on and never did. Kindness, a word of praise—I never had. [HERE IS A BIG CHANGE IN RUTH:] Now I want a home, perhaps even to be a wife. I don't know. But I want to run a house for a man. I have had enough of women and children. I frankly want to be loved and cared for. I have had enough of giving; it's time now to receive. But never would I fool with any married man.

4-14-59　　Doctor, you are right; when I decrease the dosage of Dilantin, my brain acts up . . .

Does it mean that in time I will mentally lose contact with the world of living people? Sometimes now as I buy some small article I find myself saying, "Please, Dear God, let me live just a little longer."

4-21-59   Under your care and guidance I have seen myself come to a living, breathing life—the wonder and joy of being a woman; to have no fear when a man speaks to me. And now again I feel it is God's plan: go back where I belong—in nursing. No matter how many excuses, whatever I say, I am lying—a hospital is the world I belong in. I love the aged people in the hospital. And yet tomorrow I may curse nursing and may say goodbye to it.

4-22-59   I went to the Nurses' Association and talked with a counselor. She said, "Take no more side roads." Now I feel I can go back into uniform and be myself again.

4-28-59   In the morning I found I had voided a small amount of urine in my bed, which was due probably to a slight convulsion, not big enough to wake me. [RUTH WAS PROBABLY RIGHT ABOUT THE CAUSE OF AN OCCASIONAL SLIGHT WETTING OF HER BED.]

Sometimes I feel that in my body is my brother's spirit. How to express it is this way: I am me, Ruth; but I am thinking with his brain, using his voice and saying to myself, "His driving force I have."

I will not destroy your work so that other people who suffer as I have suffered will lose hope. [AS I SAID ABOVE, RUTH WANTED HER CONFESSION TO HELP HUNDREDS OF THOUSANDS OF FELLOW SUFFERERS.]

4-29-59   Brother A. and I discussed finances. I am cashing $200 for him so he will start a bank account. But never again do we meet—and THAT I mean. [THIS IS CURIOUS, BECAUSE THE ONE PERSON IN LIFE WHOM RUTH LOVED SEEMED TO BE BROTHER A.]

Dr. Alvarez, I now realize that my father's life was hell —the nights he walked, unable to sleep. Finally, he would wake our mother, saying, "Minnie, wake up and talk to me."

He slept very little. As I look back, I am pretty sure my father, like me, had a mild epilepsy.

We children lived in hell.

These are the little incidents I have seen as Brother A. and I have been together: he is unable to wear a necktie. I asked him why, and he said, "I feel it chokes me." Brother A. does not know, and I will never tell him, why my hands jerk and jump; even sometimes now after the wonderful care you have given me. Two of my brothers drink a bit too much, but I cannot drink because if I do *I get so angry I am likely to fight someone.*

4-30-59   Now, I know why Brother A. never carries a knife, and leaves a bar as soon as someone in the place starts a fight. He fears he might, in an insane anger, kill someone. I admit that the knife I once threw at him, if it had gone home, would have pierced his heart. What was our argument? Well, he was then in charge of our finances. One day I said, "We have five cents left; let's buy some strawberries." He said, "No," and then all hell broke loose in me. [SO VERY TYPICAL OF EPILEPTIC IRRITABILITY, SHE CHASED HIM THROUGH THE HOUSE WITH A CARVING KNIFE IN HER HAND. LATER SHE WAS SO THANKFUL THAT SHE HAD NOT KILLED HIM. BUT THIS SHOWS SO CLEARLY THE DANGER THAT SOME EPILEPTICS RUN OF HURTING SOMEONE.]

I now have no fear of the hallucination voices. I sleep, or lie awake in the dark. Nowadays I can't stand a light on. I am not worried or frightened by the dark as I used to be.

5-1-59   I admit I was hell to live with at times. Lately I have been trying to get a new job, but so far, without any luck.

Now, as my handwriting changes, I see myself getting excited. In a beautiful vision in the long ago, my mother said, "Wait, Ruth, and I'll come for you." And I felt her happiness when, in a dream, she walked into your waiting room with me. Brother A. and I love each other. Yes, we are the two unmarried members of the family. So what?

5-5-59   Having my brother here to talk to is good for me. He used to stutter, and with him I too stuttered a little.

5-6-59   I realize this: from my father we children inherited this instability and fear. Also, from my mother's side, I inherited hell's own temper. Perhaps because of Father's temper he was rejected forever by his family. Twice they cast him out. On Mother's side, her father was the stern, unrelenting Puritan type. Grandmother? She and I hated each other, and my life with her was a hell on earth. She kept asking, "Why aren't you as smart as your eldest brother?"

Here is why I went into nurse's training. I thought I was in love with a young doctor who took care of our family when we were ill. My classmate straightened that out after she asked me some pointed questions. Any love for the man was soon burned out.

5-9-59   Dr. Alvarez, I can't live without some love. Without it I die slowly and surely. And people have this line, "I can't understand you," and they never will, partly because they love to talk about their own troubles and problems.

5-16-59   For me, Brother A. has been a tonic. I needed him. We were at a cafeteria; my darling set down his tray, then brought mine. *I was cared for and that was delightful.* On crossing the street he took me by the arm— me? I never heard of such a thing. He said, "If the doctor feels you can write so that others will be helped, you write." His face glowed as he told me this.

5-24-59   I often wander around in a daze, trying to make up my mind. What a joke. I know what I want when I shop, but before I buy it, I have to walk around the block, then come back.

I decided today that Brother A. is my guest; I asked him, "How about a dancing lesson for each of us?" And for me, no more lonely room or apartment. Get out into the world of amusement, or end in a mental hospital. What would my brother's life have been years ago if I had had to give up and leave him helpless, unable to walk or talk? Brother now writes well if he takes his time. He taught himself to read and write.

A knock came at my door, a man saying something. I said, "What do you want?" Again he knocked. I said, "Listen, just try to come in; I have a loaded revolver, and certainly know how to use it. So go ahead, come along." Later, I called the hotel desk to see if the clerk had seen my caller.

6-3-59   The door is now locked, and against it is a heavy ironing board. In a dream, on my bed lay the infant Jesus, sleeping so sweetly. Then in came a father, mother, and a girl about twelve years old. The father and mother were pulling a crib containing a baby, oh, so ill. The mother picked up her child; then she took a cigarette and started to smoke. Shocked I was. The mother held the cigarette to the child's lips and let him take a puff or two. Then he spurned it.

6-6-59   To this day I can hear my brothers say, when I was a girl, "Ruth is scared. She's having a nightmare." Brother A. could reach my door first, and he would put his arms around me. Then in would run Brother E, at that time my dearest, most treasured honey. Two pairs of arms, holding me so close, and the boys saying, "You are all right; we are with you." Later Brother E. would say, "A., stay with Ruth and I'll go back to bed." So A. would roll up in a blanket on top of the covers, close to me, so I was not alone. And long before I wakened, he would go back to his bed. In spite of all my hell-raising, I was loved.

6-12-59   Years ago, on leaving for a war, Brother E. wrote me, telling of his love and thanks. He told me that if he did not come back from the war, I should keep and use the money he had left with me. How I treasured that note.

6-16-59   Too bad I never learned to attract men. Too late now. But I am ready to be put out of my misery. My greatest mistake has always been, "Be honest." So I am sick, tired, and fed up.

6-17-59   Before the Dear God guided me to you, the nights I spent in bitter tears and fear. The kindness you have awakened in me: *I am a new woman.*

6-28-59   At last I have found work with a woman with two children. I am alone most of the time. Just what I wanted. Frankly, my family are now a pain in the neck to me. If we never meet, fine. We had our last argument this time, and it's permanent. From now on, I plan to enjoy myself a lot more than I did. My family have always acted as if any illness on my part is imagined. What a shock they would all have if they knew the truth. But that dies with me. [CURIOUSLY, RUTH, WITH ALL HER DESIRE TO HELP PEOPLE WITH A MILD UNRECOGNIZED EPILEPSY WITH MANY TERRIBLE FORMS OF NERVOUSNESS ONLY TWICE WAS WILLING TO HELP A BROTHER AND A NIECE, BY SENDING THEM FOR AN ELECTROENCEPHALOGRAM. THE BROTHER GOT THE TEST WHICH, AS I SAID, SHOWED EPILEPSY, BUT THE NIECE REFUSED TO SEE ME.]

My brain is calming down. My new course of beauty treatment is paying off nicely, and one of these days I shall be beautiful. The calm and quiet are doing much for me.

10-15-59   I now feel healthy and happy most of the time, and then an attack of depression may come and hit me like a bomb. It never lasts but a day or less. I fight it off and then laugh. I am satisfied.

Recently as I dozed, I heard a call, "Ruth," then I felt a slap on my face. Another night, I felt someone lying on my back.

10-20-59 Today, very dizzy—stumbling, falling against objects, frequent, slight loss of memory. I return from a "far distance" to ask what has been said. I felt I was in a grey fog.

12-3-59 I am beginning to coordinate slowly, to accept my brain storms. I realize I am a problem, but I can and do laugh.

Chapter V—1960

1-26-60   Certain music often makes me feel like dancing. Alone I may try a few steps but then I tell myself I am silly; also you are too old, or I get religious and say it is sinful to be so gay.

2-9-60   I am having spells of fear.

8-5-60   During all these months that I did not write, I was terribly depressed and ill and alone. Sometimes I wrote letters but I was too depressed to mail them. I did not even feel like coming to your office or telephoning you. But now I am getting over my depression and I am again turning my face forward. I have been through a serious change in personality. Frankly, I went to hell, and the Devil took over but good. I am now getting back to a more calm disposition.

Once I wrote my elder brother H., saying, "Once and for all, don't try to live my life for me, telling me I must go on with nursing." So he wrote and said that it's best we don't correspond; he said we get too emotional. The problems of everyday life—I couldn't always meet them well until I came to you.

8-13-60   Last night I started off into a severe seizure. How handsome the face of a young sailor in white was that appeared to me; then I saw Brother E. I jerked slightly, but came out of that, and the mist cleared quickly. My chest feels off and on as if someone hit me hard.

8-17-60   Yesterday when I went to the bank I was too confused to make a deposit.

8-31-60   Recently I read an article saying that some sleepwalkers are epileptic. Is that why I and my feeble-minded brother walked in our sleep? [IT PROBABLY WAS.]

9-15-60   Today I received a letter from my sister-in-law who was recently widowed. She asked me not to visit

her; I remind her too much of her husband. I have no desire
to set foot in that house ever again, and I shall never again
unless I get a letter first.

10-3-60   Yesterday twice my right foot jumped and
an ankle turned. Two times I had blackouts, and once I became very sleepy. I sat down half awake, with my head on
the table, and wondered, Where am I mentally?

10-6-60   As I washed dishes, I felt Brother E. standing close beside me.

10-9-60   This is the third time I changed my will,
and now it's final.

10-15-60   My mind gets distorted; I see faces or hear
a voice. Now I just laugh; I know my trouble and what it is.

Now it comes back—this memory: when I was a child
living with Grandmother she would put me into a screaming
rage. For years my face was pitted, also my hands were
wounded, after I had torn at my skin in a spell of anger; and
now I remember my mother calming me and bandaging
my hands. When Grandmother put in her two cents worth,
oh, boy, did I get mad.

If Brother H. had died before I knew you, I would never
have tried to come back; I would have gone ahead and died.
Today, I must live so that I can write this diary that will give
thousands of other nervously ill people like me the courage
to fight onward. It can be done. For the first time in my life,
I am out of prison. I will never be a fool again, giving in to
myself.

11-8-60   Yesterday was the strangest day I ever lived
in. I woke with a slight headache, and suddenly I got lost.
I was looking at the calendar, and thought the month of
November was about gone. Downtown I had the feeling that
everybody was looking so strange; I wondered if I was in an
unknown country. This is my reason for not voting; a voting
machine, you can explain it to me forever, and I won't un-

derstand it, no matter how simple it is. It's just like the weighing scales; my mind doesn't register what I see.

My Brother A., for my birthday, sent me some lovely pins and an ornament for my hair, but they made me so nervous that I just broke everything up, except one pin that I kept. [RUTH USUALLY REACTED BADLY TO ANY GIFT: IT MADE HER VERY ANGRY. SHE HATED TO FEEL "OBLIGATED" TO ANYONE.]

12-26-60   Frankly, it's wonderful to be 53 years old. I feel younger while I grow older.

I cut down on medicine for a few days. [TOO OFTEN RUTH DID THIS AND SUFFERED FOR IT.] Then my hands jerked and struck things so often and I started dreaming so much. Now I take medicine as needed. On less medicine, I became afraid—perhaps I will be out of work. But last night in my sleep I almost wet the bed. I woke up in time. I was dreaming about a little girl, telling her the floor was not a bathroom.

My brother's daughter is going to a mental clinic; she gets depressed.

Chapter VI—1961

1-17-61   During the day I have had a feeling of hysteria. I just wanted to scream, run away, quit and get out of sight.

One night, suddenly, I felt I was in New York's Grand Central Station. I never have been there; but I have seen the station in movies and television. I was speaking to a strange woman; a little girl was with her. Suddenly the child and the woman were gone.

One day I took a pan out of the oven, and suddenly, I was out, blank. I must have picked up the pan with my bare hands and put it on the stove, but how I did it I don't know. I had only a small burn on my hands. [*NOTE:* VERY FEW PATIENTS HAVE TOLD ME, AS RUTH HAS DONE, THESE TROUBLES IN THE KITCHEN OF A PERSON WITH BRIEF BLACKOUTS, OR SPELLS OF PETIT MAL.]

It's always amazing to me, the change that comes in me after I take an extra dose or two of Dilantin. Then I feel wonderful. All my problems then clear right up. I seem to be able to work with a clearer head; and I don't feel irritable and hysterical.

I am proud of one of my young nieces who is planning to go to college. She has a good brain. Her sister finished college in 3 years.

2-21-61   Your office is one place I am not afraid to come to; there I am among friends.

2-25-61   I woke up one morning with the pillows, which are usually at the foot of my bed, across the floor, so I must have had a seizure. I then felt such a change; I had an entirely different personality. I was irritable. I wanted to walk out and keep on going. It's over now, and I have myself in hand. I woke up one night, halfway out of bed, and a bit wet; I had started to void. The minute I am upset, I am so changed. What gets me is that nagging fear that perhaps I owe income tax for past years.

3-2-61   I received a letter that left me dazed and close to a heart attack. The letter is supposed to be from my brother E. The handwriting looked like his. I read very little of it; two lines were enough. It was nasty. He said he never again wanted me to visit his home; he never again wanted to see me or hear from me; also I would never have a chance to insult his wife again. For all I know, my real brother may be dead, and an imposter has taken over. I tore up the letter, feeling stunned. I wrote a short, angry note. If I get another letter, I'll send it to you, Doctor; I won't open it; my blood pressure can't take it, but I would feel better to hear what you think. From the day brother E. married—or was it him? I'll never know—it's been the same thing: a lovely letter from me, then after that, screams of rage, and his claim that he has been insulted. Why, I don't know. E. is a lone wolf; everyone has gotten hell from him. I now have one regret; I should have saved my brother's letter to read when I was calm.

3-31-61   Now I want a vacation. [A DOCTOR HAD SUGGESTED AN OPERATION TO REMOVE HER HEMORRHOIDS, AND SHE BECAME EXTREMELY UPSET.]

4-21-61   Saturday the children and I [CHILDREN OF HER EMPLOYER] are going to see a movie and have lunch. It's amazing; two little angels are living here with me. I am firm, but I try to give enough leeway so a child can think.

I was listening to radio music. Suddenly, I thought I was standing, looking at a beautiful baby with the bluest eyes, sitting on his mother's lap. I sank into darkness; I tried to come out, but was unable to. I felt my head jerk back; then it began to get lighter for me. I could see again. In spite of the medicine, I have bad dreams when I am upset. [MANY EPI-LEPTICS HAVE TOLD ME THAT EVEN WHEN THEIR DISCOMFORTS HAVE BEEN WELL UNDER CONTROL WITH DILANTIN, SOME ANNOYANCE CAN CAUSE THEM TO HAVE SPELLS OF THEIR MILD EPILEPSY.]

4-22-61 This I have learned; to stop stooping over as I walk; to hold myself erect. The world is full of cruelty when people discover your weakness.

I received a letter from brother E., saying he was sorry he had written as he did. To follow the Master, one must always be ready to forgive. So I'll write a friendly letter.

[BROTHER E.'S LETTER TO RUTH] "Dear Sis: Sorry I wrote you the rough letter; just a misunderstanding on my part. Otherwise everything same as before. My wife is wonderful and our daughter is fine. You are always welcome in our house, and we look forward to your visit. I may not be here [E. WAS IN THE MERCHANT MARINE], but our house is your house. That letter I sent you was all my fault. My wife says 'Hello,' and loves you." [THIS SHOWS THAT THE BROTHER COULD ALSO HAVE A VIOLENT TEMPER TANTRUM, WHICH HE COULD REGRET. WHENEVER I WANT TO LEARN HOW WELL AD-JUSTED A PATIENT AND HIS RELATIVES ARE, I ASK HOW HE LIKES HIS RELATIVES, AND IF HE SAYS, "THEY ARE ALL BASTARDS," I KNOW THAT THEY ARE BAD-TEMPERED AND LACKING IN SELF-CONTROL AND PROBABLY HAVE SOME SERIOUS HEREDITARY NERVOUS TROUBLE.]

4-30-61 My brain in the gynecologist's office went off duty like a flashlight, on and off. I was told to remove my clothing from the waist down, but I remembered nothing, and undressed from the waist up. The doctor said the best way to carry off a situation is with a sense of humor, and so I did.

5-6-61   I had a week of such perfect hell that I stopped all medicine. Each dose, when I took it, made me feel like I was swallowing a charge of grouchiness. I felt better when I went off medicine for almost a week. I now have started back gradually; I'm over being so irritable.

Brother E. wrote me a lovely letter again, and I wrote that next Christmas I would come out for a week. *I am fine until my brothers write. They worry so over me, and that makes me wild with rage. I know it shouldn't.*

5-7-61   Now I remember that my bladder and rectal trouble came when I was working in a hospital where, when your bladder or bowel is full, you may not be able quickly to go to the bathroom; you just have to stand there and suffer. So constipation developed. Everybody said, "Calm down; relax." But how could I? I suffered in sympathy with each sick or dying person and the family. The authorities sent me to a psychiatrist who spent all the time trying to make me confess I had been a "scarlet sister." Sexually, my body never troubled me till the menopause.

Last Thursday, my day off, was the queerest day. People looked so odd, their eyes were just immense. But I fought back my fear of them and held on to my mind. After a movie I felt better.

5-11-61   Today, Brother E. wrote; he wants to borrow $65. Was I boiling! That bitch he married is always after money. For the present, I'll just not write, and see what happens. I feel something is crooked. E. earns good money when he works. He is not lazy and he does not now drink too much. But I wrote back, "Forget me; your wife has been nothing but trouble. I have my own worries."

5-25-61   Now I realize what brought on my attacks: it was a shock. I don't know how to handle this problem, and I am even ashamed to write. Perhaps I am making a mountain out of a molehill. I told myself just to leave the job and be done. Well, it's this: the eleven-year-old boy here puzzles me. Whenever he can he likes to press his body against mine—against my back. At times he touches me in the rectal area. When he did this, I quietly said, "Stand up and behave." Next day I was on my knees, looking for vegetables; when he got down, got his head under my arm, he lay against my breast. I do wear a girdle but no brassiere. I was sick from shock—nausea hit me badly. That night, or a night later, off I went with the spells. So now I am extra careful; I allow no standing near or being touched.

5-27-61   I give away each gift I get; I cannot be bought. [THIS IS TYPICAL OF THE EXTENT TO WHICH RUTH FEARED DEPENDENCY.] I have only one gift in this house I will keep—my wristwatch. [LATER, SHE THREW THAT AWAY ANGRILY.] I more than earned it. All the other junk I threw away or gave away. My employer and I are getting along fine; I guess we took each other's measurements for the present.

5-28-61   I am back in the doghouse with my family. I sent my niece $75 as a graduation gift. But I got worried, when no letter came, and no phone call. So I called up. My sister-in-law said, "Well, J. was upset." [APPARENTLY SHE RESENTED A GIFT JUST AS RUTH DID.] The more I thought about it, the madder I got. I wrote my niece a note, saying, "Return the check and I'll never again trouble myself. We will never meet again."

6-4-61   I saw the movie *The Pleasure of His Company,* and I'm sorry I went. All I can say is this: if I had a daughter marrying a blockhead who was buying a bull on his honeymoon, I would have said, "Daughter, this is your future; if someday a cow is having a calf and you are having a baby, your husband will be out in the barn helping the cow."

6-12-61   I wonder—will I have more trouble as I get

older. Because if my future gets darker, I must now plan what to do or where to go. I don't want to be in a nursing home ever. But life looks as if I won't have much to say about it.

6-19-61　　　I can think better, but to weigh myself is still a puzzle—ounces, quarters, etc., I still don't know or remember.

I have suddenly the sharpest hot flushes. Last Thursday, my face, ears, and much of my body were on fire. The feelings came and went. The next days, my arms were also on fire. I checked my temperature; 97.6°. My feet burn, and then back comes distress into my face.

7-4-61　　　Dr. Alvarez, when I write you, I have no fear. Now I accept what I sense, or the voice that once in a while tells me, "Wear only this dress," or "Do not go there." I have learned that it's best to listen and obey. One day, when I went downtown, suddenly I felt ill, and I heard this command, "Go to church now." I did; I sat and prayed, then went on, and I was fine.

7-13-61　　　Often I hear a wife say, "I run this house." Then, when something comes up in regards to the child, the man's face may turn white. I have a temper and so I know the anger that can rise in one when a woman makes a remark like that. Men work so hard, and often for what? Children grow up, go away, or marry. Husband and wife must make the bonds closer for the long time of being together.

7-16-61　　　I could be bitter and hate each sister-in-law. But once one has felt love for the Master, one shouldn't hate anyone. Not that I can't boil like an erupting volcano. It's a year since my brother died. I sat down and wrote three of the nicest letters I could to my sisters-in-law. I know what it is to be alone. I said, "The past is over; face forward; it's now we live." God doesn't put up with people who make promises and break them, but I know if I ever have surgery, I'll die.

7-19-61   The other day it was funny; as I looked, one person became four.

8-1-61   God led me over a long, dark road to you. I feel now that He asks that I give in gratitude to poor people until my life is gone. [RUTH WRITES THE NEXT LETTERS WHILE SHE IS ON VACATION: SHE WENT TO A BIG CITY HOTEL FOR TWO WEEKS, PLANNING TO REST AND SIGHTSEE.]

After you began to wake up my brain, you told me, "You are really an attractive woman," and that cheered me no end. I went downtown today and bought a love of a little hat with a tiny, perky feather. I also got a necklace. At last I can wear things around my neck. [FOR YEARS RUTH HAD BEEN SO INTOLERANT OF CONFINEMENT THAT SHE COULD NOT EVEN STAND THE PRESSURE OF A HAT ON HER HEAD OR A STRING OF BEADS AROUND HER NECK.]

As I was leaving the bus station, across from my hotel, and had reached street level, a man put up his hand in motion to come over. He was so sad. We talked and he said I attracted him greatly because I look so much like his dead wife. He offered me the chance to be a bird in a gilded cage, with a nice apartment, money, a housekeeper, anything I might want. His wife has been dead some years. I pretended to be so innocent. I told him I could never marry. I spoke with all the gentleness and kindness I had; I don't believe in hurting people. I could see he was not well.

8-6-61   Today I found at long last that I could write to the doctor I had known once and loved [THE PSYCHIATRIST]. I did not say anything to hurt him, but I said that at long last I knew the truth. It is God's plan for me to wander up and down a long road.

8-7-61   Yesterday I had a blackout that lasted longer than anything I ever had before.

8-12-61   I used to be ashamed because I had no sex life. What was wrong? I just can't sleep with or date any man. For what? I want to be a woman in my own right. I want to be treated with courtesy. I get that.

8-25-61   I am making my funeral arrangements. I want to be sure that there are NO SERVICES. I am prepared for the hour of my death. I only pray that I will not die here and frighten the children.

My vision is triple off and on.

The last time Brother A. and I met, he noticed a kindness and a change in me, and we were able to talk peacefully.

After reading the autobiography of Margiad Evans, *A Ray of Darkness,* I had a memory: there were nights I used to worry, when, like Mrs. Evans, I thought I had harmed a child. The terror I felt! How awful if a wee one were dead because of me. But now I am so much better. [I SUGGESTED THAT RUTH READ EVANS'S BOOK TO SEE HOW INTERESTING AND HELPFUL AN HONEST LIFE STORY OF A PERSON WITH MILD EPILEPSY CAN BE TO OTHER PERSONS WITH A MILD EPILEPSY.]

9-7-61   Recently I had a fuss with my employer, but thank God that is over. But any upset takes me days to get over. I gave my nerves a workout, I realize, but I'll die before I back down in an argument I didn't start.

Here is a list of the places in which I worked:

10 years—private duty in a hospital.

3 months—in another hospital; conditions there would have made a head of a board of health jump up and down with rage.

5 years—general duty in a hospital; during the last 2 years there I was ill off and on. Everybody including the psychiatrist had a field day with me; I had sleep narcosis treatment and drugs.

8 months—general duty in another hospital, working with

nuns; fine women; but some conditions were so distressing to me that my blood pressure went way up.

4 years—night duty in a church home for infants and preschool children. The conditions were not good.

5 years—24-hour duty in a home for unmarried mothers.

2 years—in charge of nurses in a clinic for handicapped children.

Then, housework in a doctor's home. My blood pressure went up and I quit; I had too little time off.

Then, housework for a very unpleasant woman.

Somewhere I spent a summer ill, but I got well.

Now, at last, I am settled with a nice family. [THE FAMILY SHE WORKED FOR CONSISTED OF AN ABLE HUSBAND, A WIFE, AND TWO CHILDREN, A BOY AND A GIRL.]

In one nursing home there were several lesbians; I never went in for that, and I don't plan to. When two in succession approached me I fought them off.

Dr. Alvarez, when I last saw you I was having a strange spell. When you spoke, I heard you as if from a great distance; also everything seemed gray. I didn't see much; I just felt lost. Out on the street, people's eyes looked so strange—like pictures of faces in magazines that used to terrify me. When new and better brains are made, I'll order the first set.

9-10-61 I learned so much from all you have shown me so kindly, so gently. I felt when I came to you that I was a hopeless case, but what kind, I did not know. Now I have hope. Let anyone explain the voices I heard one wonderful day, the healing and lifting of a great burden as a priest blessed the congregation; my tears came and fell like a flood. Many times God must have heard me praying.

When I was a child of about seven or eight, I had a terrible shooting pain in the rectum, but I never told anyone—I took it. Weeks would pass, then suddenly I had it again, sharp and sudden. [IN SOME VERY NERVOUS PEOPLE, SUCH SEVERE RECTAL PAIN SEEMS TO ARISE IN THE BRAIN.]

Curiously, when in the evening I have a slight convulsion in my bed, next day I feel much better; more relaxed. The storm is over. From now on, if the feeling comes, I will stay in bed and have a spell.

Strange—I never received an answer to my letter to the psychiatrist I loved and lost.

9-15-61   Recently I stopped taking my medicine for a few days until I was walking in darkness irritable and just awful. Then I took more medicine, and that day I felt like an angel, calm and relaxed. Lately, I just want to walk continually; I enjoy the museums. I can't always sit quietly in a movie or even enter one; I have been having trouble with speech; I can't remember words. On my way to do something, I get lost; I start for the bathroom and forget why, or I find myself unexplainably in the hall.

9-16-61   Last night I had a terrifying experience. Suddenly all began to go black, and a tall figure appeared. Now that I am over the shock, I'll try to describe what happened. I was so frightened I wanted to scream. The man was dressed in black leather garments; his face gave me a terror I can't describe. The expression was so dark, so full of bitterness and hate. But then a beautiful garden appeared and I fell asleep. This morning I am fine.

9-18-61   I am afraid to open a window and look out; I don't trust windows that are several stories up; I might jerk, and then Goodbye.

9-20-61   I am in a hell of a temper. I feel sorry for the husband here where I work. Working for a damned fussy woman is something I would wish on my worst enemy. Hell will freeze over before any damned bitch walks over me.

This woman loves to dominate, but I too have to have my say. And I do, job or no job.

9-21-61   Yesterday, the little girl spoke so loud I covered my ears. For some reason, it feels as if my head is being squeezed together. [MANY EPILEPTICS ARE VERY DISTRESSED BY LOUD NOISES.]

9-25-61   Once and for all, I returned a watch that was given me. I just can't stand the feelings associated with a gift. I refused it and said, "The hell with it. I will buy my own, and that is that." Gifts—I have had it. NEVER another gift. I hate them. [HER NICE EMPLOYER HAD GIVEN HER A WRIST WATCH. USUALLY SHE WAS ON HIS SIDE DURING HIS ROWS WITH HIS WIFE.]

I don't know really what it is, but I am fighting a marked change in my personality. I don't ever *want* to be the devil to live with. I do feel rich warmth, and love is coming back. I want to be a happy woman, not one buried in tragedy.

10-1-61   Dr. Alvarez, I want to go to the Aleutian Islands. It is strange how Alaska calls me. I must go. I will love a quiet world with no radio, no newspapers, but great scenery, volcanoes, nature as God created it. It offers what I want—the peace of God—and no husbands in my life. I inherited from my father the wanderlust.

10-7-61   I lay in bed asleep, and heard some sounds like a whistle; I felt that a young man pinched me. Hell's fires flamed in me; I slapped his face, then I looked at him; he stood with his eyes closed. I was worried; did I kill him? Then I woke up; what a relief!

10-19-61   I can't take teasing from my employer; teasing I don't understand. I told her that once a doctor who teased me almost got a knife between his eyes. When I say, "Hands off of me," I mean just that. The doctor teased me once too often. These damned women—angels one time, devils from hell the next time.

10-21-61   I wish someone would come along and give me a million dollars, as it happens on television. All of you dear people would be my guests, and we'd go on a vacation.

10-27-61   Today I told my employer I have had more than enough of her nagging and fussing. No bitch like this is going to break my heart. It's hell—the fussing and nagging; I can't take it like I used to; these days I talk back.

11-1-61   I feel as if a hurricane hit me. Today I was stiff as a board. I can't stand these damn arguments. This damned woman—tonight, another battle. Over what?

[LATER] Peace again. We both laugh, sooner or later. This woman is a liar and we'd better part. I hope this will be the last damned woman I ever work for.

11-21-61   Dr. Alvarez, you never lay down the law; you expect and trust me to stand on my own two feet. And that to me is like being given a million dollars, tax free. [THIS IS SO TYPICAL OF RUTH'S GREAT NEED FOR FREEDOM AND INDEPENDENCE.]

11-26-61   I am lucky I have my shaking spells in my sleep. I can hold myself together all day. When I lived with Rose, she saw me have one of my attacks in my sleep; she left me alone and I came out of it. I slept on and never knew until later what had taken place.

I see now why we women can't be presidents. Menstrual periods can make a woman haywire. I know that those were the times when nothing was right within me.

12-3-61   Today, as I suddenly for a while could not speak, I knew what my little brother had suffered during the years when he stuttered, and had trouble talking.

12-6-61   You, Doctor, and your two secretaries, have all done so much for me. After all the wonderful help and guidance you have given me. Always I receive so much kindness from you and I so appreciate your acceptance of me the way I am.

Back east—it is a terrible memory; a nurse, with her eyes blazing, choking me and telling me I must be quiet. I screamed; I guess I was drugged, excited. I don't know. I only remember a night filled with terror. I had fainted the third time on duty, and some idiot called the superintendent of nurses. What with being rushed to a room, lying on a cart, and listening to the women raving, I remember a pillowcase being put over my head; I was nude; I heard someone say, "We can't keep a gown on her." I then fought nurses and interns; there were six people trying to control me; I got to the window several times to jump out. [SOME EPILEPTICS HAVE BRIEF SPELLS OF SUCH PSYCHOSIS. RUTH HAD A TERRIBLE ONE ONCE WHEN SHE BROKE HER ANKLE AND WAS TAKEN TO A HOSPITAL.]

Now all the hell is over; I am cared for, but with the freedom to go to a doctor only when I feel it's needed.

12-11-61 I promised God that I would never forget others, and whatever I can do to help, I'll be more than happy to do. If you wish to arrange my diary in book form, go ahead. But will you mind if I never want to read about myself? It's the past. I am in the present. What I much want is that many others who suffer like me can be helped.

The first time I wanted to scream I had sense enough to leave the table where I was sitting with other nurses, and to go out of doors. No one noticed me.

12-19-61 One of my brothers introduced me to a charming man, hoping that I might fall in love with him, but I couldn't hurt the feelings of an innocent person; I just was not interested. If I were a woman who could really care for a man, nothing would keep me from it.

12-28-61 I still don't understand about my Brother E. But I will take his name out of my will. He and Brother A. met, and A. was invited to dinner; later he was told, "Never come back." Each sister-in-law has closed the door also against me.

Chapter VII—1962

1-4-62   It's wonderful to feel so well that when a spell is over I can quickly forget it. Now I can sometimes tell that a spell is coming; I feel nervous, irritable, and wishing I was dead. And then I think of what you told me; *the good part of my brain will carry me through.* I tell myself that, and then I feel much better.

1-8-62   In September I sail on the mail boat to the Aleutian Islands. I want to see the country God created.

1-18-62   I am a strange woman. I tend to be either deliriously happy, walking on the clouds, or so depressed that I think suicide would be the best thing. Years ago I had to earn a living for me and for my two youngest brothers. Even then, days could come when I just had to leave my job. Sometimes it was to care for a sick brother. Today if I have temper trouble with someone, I just say, "My blood pressure is up," and I get kindness and sympathy.

Today I was confused for hours. It started when I tried to figure out a card for the girls. This is me; I can talk and laugh, but later my mind goes blank. I feel I must show that I want to be like other people, not the person I have been.

Dr. Alvarez, it is so remarkable, since taking Dilantin I experience emotions I never knew before in my life. Now I can give my family a kiss and a hug; and can act with warmth and affection. My dentist, bless him, had tears in his eyes, when he spoke about the great change in me for the better—looking well and self-assured. In this home when I work I watch the marriage of the man and his wife. To me such a marriage would be hell. One frown, and I would kill the guy. And sometimes, when I go to bed, I have that old fear—that I might harm someone and not know it.

1-21-62   Once or twice in the past I wanted to kill

115

the nurse who was trying to hold me down in bed. The doctor had given me morphine, but that drug causes the softest voice or slightest noise to be magnified so loud that I want to escape. I have been told that I never hush up when I've been given the drug. [I HAVE SEEN MANY SUCH HIGHLY NERVOUS PERSONS WHO ARE VIOLENTLY STIMU-LATED BY A SEDATIVE DRUG.] And before I came to you—well, I can say I do feel sorry for those doctors who had me on their hands. No one could help me, partly because no one understood me.

1-25-62   In a steak house a young man asked if he could share my table. We talked a little. He was nervous and jumpy as a cat—after having had a fight with his mistress. No one's life is easy. I just sat calmly and he left. Poor man; it's hell. The Devil drives, and I often wonder—where?

Nuns are strange people; they are friendly, but they can suddenly change.

1-26-62   Sometimes my foot catches a leg of a table or chair. I don't know; it just happens, and then I am likely to fall heavily. Today, I laughed all day.

2-11-62   The boy [THE SON OF RUTH'S EM-PLOYER] again rested his hands on my breasts. I stepped back. For a long time this has not happened. But his mother saw this action. Had the father been around, hell would have broken loose. I don't like it, and yet if I tried to explain that to the boy when he and I are alone—well, children just pull down a shade. When does one start teaching a boy manners?

2-21-62   I saw the movie *King of Kings* Sunday, and I was impressed. It was all the way I imagined Jesus would look—his eyes, so clear, serene, and deep into one's soul he looked. There were two scenes I could not watch—the killing of John the Baptist, and the crucifixion. I couldn't watch, and I had to hold on tight to myself not to have a seizure. The storms in one's brain are swift. I know I can't ever again see a picture like it; it's best not to. But it was all as I had imagined it through the years.

Sunday I had three children here. The boy put on an act; he said he had to eat alone, and gave me directions thus and so. I exploded quite well. From children I take no orders; I give them. So all got calm. I am in charge. I put the card table up and the children watched television, ate dinner together, and were no trouble. The boy carried the dishes out. I didn't even ask him to. I am firm; my nurse's training is a big help. I prefer to drop dead from a good dose of anger than to take being walked over.

3-3-62   Right now I am in a perfect rage. This damned woman is so afraid I will eat a meal! She bought some beef and I said I would prepare it for dinner for the children and myself. Fine; I put it on about 4 P.M. I like meat hard enough to chew. Not in strings. But hell broke loose. I took the damned meat and put it right in the refrigerator. I went and ate some dinner out, but not too much. I told Mrs. S. I have my way, she has hers. But in the future, no meat do I cook or serve. So it's back in the oven to get done. I hope to hell she chokes on it. I never saw such a damned woman. Her husband is home, and as usual, he kept quiet. I like him; he is always nice. During the depression of 1929 I knew real hunger. Hence, an argument over food makes me sick.

I am on the lookout for a new job.

I saw the movie *The Children's Hour* [A PLAY BY LIL-LIAN HELLMAN, IN WHICH THE CHILDREN IN A PRIVATE SCHOOL STARTED A SCANDAL ABOUT THE HEADMISTRESSES BEING LESBIANS]. I just hate being touched by man or woman. But I have enough emotions to have loved deeply, and sincerely, twice. It was a man each time. So I never get excited and feel abnormal. The last time I visited my classmate she asked me to rub her legs. I used to do that and think nothing of it. Well, her daughter, of high school age, came to the door; the look of shock on her face! And so, evil was seen where none existed.

Once a lesbian student nurse and I really had it. We were roommates. A more beautiful girl I have never seen. Her actions—I reported them, and got the blame. Well, before I was through I got an apology.

All my life I thought I was queer, mentally ill, and I had no hope. And then you, Dr. Alvarez, opened doors that led me back to health.

In your latest book, you healed a lot of suffering. But there were so many things I could not understand. Why did I act the way I did, knowing I was raising hell? Why couldn't I stop? Years ago I fainted and the nurses thought I had put on an act. Now I know it was a slight epileptic storm.

3-10-62   Well, all is peace again after the terrible fight with Mrs. S. I told her that I hate to fight, and I can't take it. I had started swearing, which usually I don't do anymore.

3-15-62   Each time now when I get ready to fuss, I remember what you said: "How much of a bill are you ready to pay for a row?" That works like a charm. I calm down and laugh.

I can't stand reading or thinking of anyone dying in the electric chair. I feel a sense of terror. The living suffer hell over and over. Who gains? I try to keep calm and not to think.

3-29-62   My niece and I had a good talk. She and her mother are not getting along. I told her, "Raise hell and be done. It will do you both good." I said something about her father, my dead brother, and she choked up and left the room. Several times we talked, I lost my mental way. The thread snapped. Interestingly, she told me that this snapping has also happened to her!

5-2-62   I told my employer one day when she fussed about her husband, "Had God given me a husband as good and kind as yours, I would kiss the ground he walked on."

5-6-62   My niece, since she left college, has not been herself. She tried suicide and she is now going to a mental clinic. [THIS GIRL APPARENTLY HAD AN EQUIV-ALENT OF THE NERVOUS ILLNESS THAT GAVE RUTH HER TROUBLES. ANOTHER ONE OF RUTH'S NIECES HAD A PSYCHOSIS.]

Dr. Alvarez, the tears for others have dried up. I just can't suffer anymore. I love the girl, but now I am letting her live her own life. And now, when my niece said, "For seconds I lose my train of thought," there was the answer. [SHE PROBABLY HAD HER AUNT'S PETIT MAL.] Help is needed, but you can't make some people believe that their condition is serious.

5-14-62   I had an eye checkup and the doctor told me that feeling irritable as I get, with loss of memory, double vision or seeing two or three people, I could have a brain disturbance, perhaps a slight hemorrhage. [AS THOUSANDS OF PATIENTS DO, RUTH DID NOT TELL THE DOC-TOR OF HER MILD EPILEPSY.]

5-15-62   I can imagine the trouble you have getting your doctor friends to believe that a patient can have epilepsy without a fall and a convulsion. Many of my spells start with my feet wrapping around each other or some object. Head-ache on awakening. Loss of memory, more than usual. Trem-ors in one or both hands and arms. Dropping things; hands just let go. Irritable—hell to keep calm and not get upset. After my spell I am fine.

5-24-62   Today I was disturbed. I was angered be-cause my sister-in-law wouldn't let my niece come to see you and see if she has what I have. As a result I had frequency of urination and some bleeding. When I get excited or upset, I can urinate every two minutes. On my day off, I have no urinary frequency at all. It's amazing.

My mother's father was very religious and very studious, but curiously, his son was not interested in education. Mother had a very good education. When she wanted to come to the United States her father said, "Not my daughter." But my mother could stand up for herself and go places on her own. So she came to the United States and got a job in a shirt-waist factory. She saved her money and later sent for her father and brother and bought her parents a home. The dislike between my father and his father was terrible! *My aunt became so queer that her husband left her.* He came and stayed with us. My father's mother had hell's own temper.

The temper I have is the most honest inheritance anyone ever got. It's strange that my brothers never swore or raised hell. My mother loved people and she had friends. Children, birds, flowers—all loved her.

All through the years my family had much to do with making me so fearful. Only my youngest brother has been close, helpful and loving.

Doctor, you put me on a sunlit road. But frankly I am now worried about being an epileptic. Should my employer ever learn what is wrong with me, I would never again be able to get work in this city; she would blacklist me. She once admitted that she had looked up my record as a registered nurse, but my old hospital manager said that my record was excellent.

6-21-62   I'll go back to the beginning, about how I got to be so strange. As a child I was a little mouse, but very observant. I knew my parents were worried about me. I was a frightened, shy little girl, who could raise hell too.

Later, I was a student nurse. One night I was sick, knocked out, miserable, crying, and thinking about Mother. Suddenly I heard a soft noise; the wall of the room rolled away and there was a beautiful valley between mountains. Mother was there, robed in white, with two lovely white wings. She was so beautiful; I can see her now, with her hands held out. I ran so quick, but Mama said, "Ruth, go back; someday I will come for you. Care for the two youngest boys." Then there was only a wall.

7-5-62 One nice thing about an attractive young man; the air gets filled with sparkles, and I enjoy myself.

All of us in my family have this in common; we do best alone; we can't be guided, pushed or pulled. Doctor, all the hell I went through to reach you makes me appreciate you all the more today. I live now. There is plenty of romance in my system. Imagination is a great gift.

7-31-62 My bladder fills up, becoming very large; to void, I must stand and lean over. At night after lying down, the bladder appears to go back in position somewhat. No pain, but retention starts. My worry is that the bladder fills, stays outside of my body most of the time. If I didn't have this hernia I wouldn't worry. [PERHAPS WHAT SHE HAD CORRESPONDED TO THE GROIN RUPTURES HER THREE BROTHERS HAD.]

8-15-62 Dr. Alvarez, I know that for me surgery is dangerous mentally. I can fight for life if I am conscious, but drugged or in pain, I doubt if mentally I would make a good fight. [THIS TURNED OUT TO BE SO CORRECT. LATER, WHEN RUTH SPRAINED HER ANKLE AND HAD TO BE KEPT IN BED IN A HOSPITAL SHE BECAME VIOLENT AND PSYCHOTIC.] All of you in your office have reached out to give me so much. God guided me to you and I won't now disgrace you.

9-2-62 One time in my life, I would like to have said, "My husband can take care of me." But I hated to think of giving up my freedom. But then again, if he comes along, why not say yes? I do get fed up with this lonely life.

9-22-62   It's strange; when I come to see you, I feel great.

10-28-62   I keep wondering if the man who wrote me, "Never return," is really my brother, Brother A., and I don't plan ever to go to see him again. I have a post office box number and I am careful who gets my phone number. [SHE WAS A BIT PARANOIAC.]

10-29-62   There came an ugly letter from Brother E. with a threat that if ever we meet I will be dealt with. Somebody is crazy.

11-15-62   If Brother E. is alive I doubt if he writes the letters I receive. From now on I plan not to read them and to be done. Once brothers H. and E. had a big fuss over the phone. Later E. wrote, "Why do you give my wife money? I work and support her." [THESE VIOLENT CLASHES BETWEEN RUTH, HER PARENTS, GRANDPARENTS, AUNT AND BROTHERS SUGGEST THAT THEY ALL SHARED THE INHERITANCE OF BAD TEMPER AND A CURIOUS NERVOUS SYSTEM.]

12-19-62   I am fighting, raising hell at bitter cost to myself. You cannot buy love and kindness with gifts; I can take things only so long, then like water bursting out of a damn, I explode. All of us have the right to be different.

12-27-62   My mind now goes back to the time seven years ago when you said to me words that are engraved on my mind and heart: "I can help you; you are a brave woman; I much admire the brave way in which, in spite of so much suffering, you have kept working hard to help people." I was healed then. A flame of hope was lit and I knew I could face anything.

Chapter VIII—1963

1-7-63   I believed no doctor until I came to you. Actually I always had felt that I had more than "just upset nerves," and you found that I was so right. Now I have a feeling of confidence.

1-13-63   I have noticed that in each month I have spells when I start to fall, and then my speech gets mixed up.

2-14-63   Thank you for not destroying my world of loveliness—with imagination, perception and warmth; you encouraged me. Psychiatry for me used to be a land of fear.

I have been having the strangest dreams lately. One night it was babies and more babies. Last night I dreamed the Madonna came, robed in black. Her face was so sad. Then I saw Queen Elizabeth and Prince Philip standing on a stage; her face was so sad, Prince Philip was calm, unsmiling. The Queen bent down and petted a small baby leopard. I was worried.

3-7-63   I must not turn back—I think of what you said, "Do it for *me*."

Today I purchased my first television set. I feel a need to know more about the outside world, so I decided to grow out, to watch world events, and to hear good music. It is not a luxury, but a necessity. I am excited, but was I foolish to buy it? I won't enjoy a nickel when I'm dead. I am getting older and hungrier for more contacts with the world. I could die mentally in this house doing housework.

8-3-63   [APPARENTLY SHE WENT THROUGH ANOTHER LONG PERIOD OF DEPRESSION, DURING WHICH SHE DID NOT WRITE ANY LETTERS. WHEN NEXT I HEARD FROM HER, SHE WAS IN THE HOSPITAL AFTER HAVING BADLY FRACTURED HER ANKLE IN A FALL. IN THE STRESS OF THE SITUA-

TION, AND BECAUSE ALL HER ANTI-CONVULSIVE MEDICINE WAS TAKEN FROM HER, SHE BECAME PSYCHOTIC AND VIOLENT.] Thank you and the girls for the lovely flowers.

This morning I had two severe seizures. I tried hard to behave, but pain and lack of sleep did me in. Once I started fighting, I so wanted to get out of bed. I am sorry; I know I caused the doctors much wastage of time. But the spell came on me so quickly. Honestly and sincerely—I love all of you dearly.

8-4-63 At 3 A.M. I broke loose, raising hell. Suddenly I saw three small, glowing bulbs and I sank into bottomless darkness. Later, I screamed. I try to behave. I feel that as soon as I am sent home and am on my own, I'll be O.K. I am not a patient that submits well to being cared for. Also, I would like to stop taking up needed space in a hospital bed. The longer the doctors have to wait for me to behave, the worse it is for all of us. In my case, the wisest thing the doctors could do would be to put me to work quickly.

These seizures give me great relief. But I feel sorry for the poor people who must put up with me. It took five people to put me in bed when I was admitted.

8-5-63 The longer I am kept in bed, the sooner I will die of a seizure. I feel so bad because I am nothing but trouble. I received the kindest and most understanding care, but an overly independent person like myself just can't take it. Do forgive me; I am a problem and getting worse. During the night I tried to get out of bed several times. I can be good just so long, and then I can't take any more. I can't help what I do.

8-13-63 I have been such a pain to my doctors and my roommate. At night I go crazy and I don't sleep. It's the nights that are a terror to me. I wish I was dead. My pride is hurt that I have to be here.

8-24-63 I have not been in my right mind all this time.

8-25-63 Yesterday I left the hospital, using a walker.

8-26-63 I can laugh again, and I feel like singing. I now have no pain, but I am in terror wondering if I will have to go back for more surgery.

8-27-63 My heart broke in a long-ago bitter hour. How cold the stars shone that night. For you I carry on. I will try to put away the thought that I might grow old and dependent. I envy my dead brothers, suddenly gone. Why not me? I must live, since I am here, because I love my employer's children, and they love me so dearly. [IT TELLS MUCH OF RUTH'S GOOD SIDE, THAT THE CHILDREN LOVED HER.]

I am getting stronger; my mistress and I had one hell of a good fight. It helped me a lot—I needed it. The Devil and I raised hell in the hospital. I felt sorry for the nurses worrying so because I wear no nightgown. I am a nudist, and that is that.

8-31-63 I don't want to marry anybody, but I may have to. When I am well, I must find a Texas millionaire and marry him. But no; I'd better not. I wouldn't know how to be wife to a millionaire. You are all invited to the wedding. If I marry, as soon as I get the oil well, I'll get a divorce and be free again. No alimony; I'll earn my own living.

I am happy to be out of the hospital. I am sick of sick people. Trouble, tears, I have had it.

9-3-63 My mistress and I have had our last fight. I can't take them any more. But leave? Let her throw me out. I stay. There is somehow, someplace, a bit of the fighting Irish in me.

9-8-63 I am so ashamed I could crawl into a hole and pull the sand over me. I am ashamed that in the hospital I threatened to end my own life. To hurt you after all that you have done to help me—no, I never will threaten that again. How can I ever face you again, having acted like a spoiled child?

[RUTH WROTE THIS FOLLOWING TO THE GIRLS IN THE OFFICE.] Dear girls; it's a pleasure to come to your office. It's strange. I am showered with blessings—I know it. I love all of you dearly, and to be told by you that I am beautiful—my mirror never talks like that. Is it wrong to enjoy all of your dear attentions?

9-25-63   My Brother A. phoned me. He was sent to a doctor, and spent three days in a hospital. He had brain wave tests, and was told that he could have a convulsion at any time. He is on anti-convulsive medication. If God wills, in the spring, Brother A. and I will meet. He is all I have to love.

Friday evening as I was washing dishes, in my mind I saw a group of angels. Their beautiful white wings, a shining light on their faces, their smiles—I just enjoyed seeing them, and out in front stood my brother who died, his arms outstretched, a smile on his face.

Then yesterday a tornado hit my brain. Storms—I had them. But I fought them off. Today I am calm and relaxed.

9-26-63   I can't help it; I am terrified when people get angry or upset. The most glorious hour in my life will be my death. I am glad I feel that one birthday more will come and then it's over. Before I die, in this house as I work there is going to be more kindness and less faultfinding.

9-28-63   I keep wanting to take my cast off and be on my own. But I can hear you say, "I wouldn't do that if I were you." No, I won't take the cast off. But I am changed in personality, no doubt about it. I didn't believe Eve had three faces; well, I think differently now: I know now I have two faces.

10-3-63   Please don't worry; I know I rave, but now

I am back to being me. I am showing you all sides of my personality. If this helps others, I will feel better. But sincerely, no word is ever written here that is not true.

10-28-63   You'll never know the joy of life until you have faced death often enough and have had to come back to life.

I sense that the day I leave this job, the lady of the house will breathe a sigh of relief. But my heart tells me to stay. I know I am a problem. The older I get, the more trouble I am.

11-4-63   The cast came off yesterday, and again I can walk. I can walk up and down steps. I feel well and do fine as long as I am left alone.

11-15-63   Now I have no desire to live or to give a damn. In all the years I have come as your patient, it has been encouragement that I received. But with all the hell I have with the orthopedist, I have never felt more alone. I'll be damned if I'll go back to the hospital. I wrote to my orthopedic surgeon and told him that I couldn't stand meeting him again. I am in the sunlight and refuse to go back into the darkness. All this care and fuss—I never asked for it.

11-17-63   I fear I am too much trouble to you. I realize that you never laugh at me. When the time comes and God gives me freedom, don't be sorry. You have given me riches that others search for all their life and do not find. I just have no desire to pretend any longer. No one will know how often I am in pain; others have it worse.

11-18-63   What has happened? Wherever I turn, it's hell in my ankle. Today I called the orthopedist to arrange for an x-ray study at the hospital. Jokingly I said, "I can walk as well as ever," and he boiled up with rage. What have I done to the man? He says I can't wear an ace bandage. But you should have seen my leg and ankle. Swollen out of sight.

I seem to be in a world that suddenly I can't understand.

Was I to blame at the hospital for being so ill? One week lost out of my life. Let the surgeon rave. I won't listen. One half of me is gone, and the rest of me I pretend is alive. Frankly, I remember very little of the accident. [RUTH MAY HAVE BROKEN HER ANKLE WHEN SHE FELL IN A CONVULSION.]

11-22-63   Today in this country the children are in charge. I was so angry one day at the children here where I work that I said, "Fine; only in America do we worship children, and neglect reality in living."

Men give me a pain.

A damned good fight would clear the air sometimes. People should do it, even if they kill each other. When I am angry, you hear me in this house; I will face the problem. This silent business is no good. If the children decide to boss me around, it won't work. I am in charge, not them.

11-30-63   All I can think of is, I CAN WALK. Nothing else seems to matter. Hanged if I will have any physiotherapy for my ankle!

Chapter IX—1964

1-2-64   Dr. Alvarez, thank you for your kindness; I no longer expect anything from anyone. I certainly had the loveliest Christmas gift: two feet to walk on, and now I feel fine.

1-10-64   The woman I work for is thinking of getting a divorce. She says that if the situation gets too bad, she will take the children and leave, and she wants me to go along. We are sitting on a powder keg. Once I would have run. Now, I settle one problem at a time.

[LATER.] Next week, I go to a hotel.

1-12-64   I feel a sense of relief, paying my own bills. [RUTH WAS SO INDEPENDENT AND IDEALISTIC THAT SHE DID NOT USE HER HEALTH INSURANCE TO COVER HER HOSPITAL AND DOCTOR BILLS WHEN SHE BROKE HER ANKLE. SHE HAD THE IDEA THAT IF SHE REFUSED TO ACCEPT MONEY FROM THE INSURANCE COMPANY, THAT MONEY WOULD BE USED FOR OTHER PEOPLE MORE NEEDY THAN SHE WAS.]

1-17-64   My two younger brothers decided never again to have me in their life. I left E. nothing in my will. If he is my real brother. I helped those two brothers start out in the world. When Brother A. was alone, I loaned him money. Now, I will give to charities as I can.

During autopsy, any part of my body to be used for study is O.K.

1-18-64   Last night, as I was on the edge of sleep, I heard my name called in terror. I realized that it was in my mind, and took two capsules of Dilantin.

Dr. Alvarez, you will say I speak strangely. But if I ever again enter a hospital, I won't be back. I don't even plan to live any more. My mind is made up, firm, once and for all. I don't plan suicide or anything, but events shaping up look bad. When all is over, I'll have a story to tell about extrasensory perception. I broke my ankle for a reason—I see it now.

1-23-64 This letter will sound like the end of the world a-coming. Thanks for all your kindness, and the courage you give me. I feel better already, writing you. Life is not smooth, it is an adventure, but until people learn that the council table is best, we will have war. And perhaps someday we can put those in charge in the battle line, and a lesson will be learned. When they come back from hell, it will be with understanding, and the feeling of people's rights. Hate, ugliness, but also loving kindness, pity, understanding. Another lesson to learn: people must learn to stand up with pride.

1-25-64 The divorce will go on quietly. But my employer thanked me for standing by her. What else can I do? I have been living in fear that a war would break out here. It's a relief to be off the powder keg for the present. I will settle all my affairs and see my lawyer. I feel owned.

1-26-64 I think about seeing the orthopedist again about my ankle, but I get terrified with him. How in heaven's name do I collect so many strange men in my life? I don't want anyone—I just want freedom: the chance to decide when I go to the doctor and when not. As you can see, any common sense I once had is gone.

1-27-64 The woman I work for doesn't realize that life alone can be like hell.

I'll stay on here and see what the effect is on me. I decided that if all is quiet, I'll stay till June. Happiness is a gift like a precious gem; you hold it only at times, not always. This place has almost broken me, but I am up again. I won't be knocked down. And I won't leave the children until I know they are safe.

[RUTH DID NOT WRITE FOR MANY MONTHS. THEN IN SEPTEMBER, SHE WROTE TO DOROTHY, MY SECRETARY.]

9-9-64 Dorothy: this is why I am afraid of a hospital. Once in, you have no rights. And I am always terrified for fear I will find myself in a mental hospital. The time has come for me to get back to being me—alive and cheerful.

Dorothy, whenever Dr. Alvarez gets too busy and tired, please take care of him. He has taught me how to walk forward.

9-11-64 Karen [RUTH'S EMPLOYER'S LITTLE GIRL], bless her; for her I must live. I do. I want this child to have a good life. The girl's grandmother brings the Devil with her. She told her grandson, "Eat this, eat that." He is eleven. Then Grandma started on me, and I got blazing angry. I had had two days of this old she-devil, so I raised hell. I told my employer either I am in charge or I leave. The children and I get along well alone. I speak and they listen. I never have to scream.

This upset distressed me, but now I feel better again.

Dr. Alvarez, how can you put up with me? But my heart speaks; I live now and I laugh now. I felt long ago that my spirit left my body, wandered, and I felt it return to the body on my bed. I cannot go on without my Dilantin. Without it, fear hits me like a brick.

11-16-64 [RUTH WROTE THIS LETTER TO DOROTHY AND CAROLYN.] I am writing my friends, so here's a line to both of you. I may not be back to you for a long time.

12-17-64 [RUTH APPARENTLY HAD FELT HER HEALTH GETTING WORSE, AND WHEN SHE

TELEPHONED MY OFFICE SHE SPOKE WITH DIFFI-
CULTY, INDICATING THAT SHE HAD HAD A FAIR-
LY SEVERE STROKE, INVOLVING LARGELY HER
THROAT.] My speech problem started about one month
ago. This week, swallowing is a problem. Food gets so far,
and then I have to drink water or hot liquid to help me
swallow. Water drains out of my nose, and I spill liquids as
I drink. Since last evening, my face and lips have been puffy.
I am very sleepy at times—too tired to stand up. My arms are
hard to raise. Lying down brings relief. I have been doing
my work.

12-28-64   I hate to ask time off from work; I get
along quietly in the house. I don't feel nervous, and my
spirits are not depressed, but I have a problem speaking. My
face gets stiff, my tongue feels tight and no one can understand me. I can see well, my hands can hold an iron. I will be
all right. I wait, my speech clears; I'll come out of this. Dr.
Alvarez, thanks for your kindness. I am sorry, but I must
get over being so tired at times. I don't want to go out and
fall down. I am all right, and I'll be back.

Chapter X—1965

1-13-65 [THIS LETTER CAME FROM THE HOS-PITAL, WHERE RUTH WAS TAKEN WHEN SHE BE-CAME TOO WEAK AND INCAPACITATED FROM THE EFFECTS OF THE BIG STROKE TO TAKE CARE OF HERSELF.]

I certainly was starving. But now my throat feels fine; my voice is improving. I talk as little as possible. Fluid pours out of both nostrils at least once a day, during meals. I am fine, and can't put into words my thanks for everyone's help and kindness. I am now able to swallow baby foods and liquids. I can speak occasionally. I feel well rested and alert, and am out of bed most of the day, reading a good book.

Dr. Alvarez, in a way I sensed my future. One night I felt the time was coming, and I should not plan a vacation. I should have realized this stroke was coming on; twice I choked—bread and meat caught in my throat; and my speech became thick. My tongue looked as if it were cut in ribbons and it burned almost continually. I had restless nights when I couldn't sleep. The morning it began in earnest, and I got so confused I couldn't think at all.

All is clearing up now. I am up in a chair. I drank for the first time normally, one half glass of orange juice. Did it taste good! I had a nasal feeding and I feel stronger. The treatment is nothing to fuss about—as long as I am not drugged, I'll cooperate.

[LATER.] Speech and food do not agree with each other. Something happens in my throat; I feel my Dilantin capsule floating around in back of my throat. I get the medicine down; if it comes up I wait and try again. I cough and choke so much.

Last night I had a seizure—I was dozing, and suddenly,

big yellow leaves pressed over my face. My head jerked back and that was all. I'll be all right; I am not worried. The doctor here is so kind and concerned. I am trying to get well real quick.

Each morning I water my precious gift, the beautiful plant your secretaries sent—and I give it a big hug and a kiss. Flowers need love—lots of it.

1-14-65   I get fed by tube by the nicest young doctors. But why all the special attention? I plan to be out soon.

1-15-65   Yesterday I had two seizures. I bathed myself in the bathroom and it wore me out. In one seizure, the room became dark. I felt sleepy, then there came visions of attractive children, flowers, scenery; I began twitching, jerking—my mouth, face, lips, then all over, completely. It left me sick.

In the second seizure, I found my arms were stiff, and then, a little later, holding medicine and water, I could not extend my arms. I fell back, trying to raise up in bed three times. Then everywhere were dark clouds, colors spinning, roaring in my ears. Cold in my feet and legs to my knees. Tingling in my left side, face, both hands, both feet. I can't remember if I screamed or moved about; then numbness cleared from my toes, both feet, the little finger in my left hand. [AS USUAL, WHEN RUTH WAS IN THE HOSPITAL, THE DOCTORS DID NOT GIVE HER THE NECESSARY ANTI-CONVULSIVE DRUGS.]

1-20-65   Now, all I can think of is, "How soon can I be free?" But before long, I'll be coming into your office, alive as usual.

1-21-65   Glory be! I am discharged. I feel fine. I realize that I was starting on this trouble slowly, when a while ago I could not button my blouse in back.

1-26-65   I am having some kind of spasms; my jaws

get stiff, and getting food down in not easy. But I am working at it. Last evening I could not close my teeth together. As usual, I can't talk well after eating.

The woman I work for says that this is my home, and I am free to stay here. I feel bad accepting help instead of standing on my own feet. I will be damned if I will give up. I will get well or drop dead. No one is going to say I was a coward and just gave up. If the story of what I experience can help others, than I am richly rewarded.

I am up and around; I will earn my food somehow.

Life can be a brutal reality. I keep quiet; I can dress, look neat, keep my room clean; I iron, and I wash dishes. I just keep quiet until my voice gets clear. I certainly feel as a bird chained to earth after knowing the glorious freedom of flying far up in the sky. This is a test, a time to accept and bow to HIS will, not mine.

Dr. Alvarez, this is my worry: I am alone. Am I taking advantage of my employer's home and kindness? Would it be best for me to find a home and give up working? What is my future? How soon can I expect more strokes? I must plan now. I know you expect me to fight on.

One night at the hospital I felt pretty well downed. And I felt someone stood by my bed, a kind hand was on my forehead. I felt at peace. If God gives me a release, I will be happy. I want to know the truth; in that way I can pick up my burden and walk. I have fought back plenty and often.

1-28-65 Dr. Alvarez, your letter was food and drink to me. I'm cured already. I am afraid of strange doctors. I always feel they size me up as a mental case.

The spasm with my jaws is lessening; I can take liquids occasionally, and the strength I have is amazing. I feel cheered up since I got up and set the table. I can be useful.

My employer says that even if I do nothing but help with the children, it is enough. I refuse to accept a paycheck from her.

I do get nervous when I can't swallow. But I will adjust myself; I am lucky that my arm and legs work. But I can't talk well.

1-29-65   My jaws are relaxing, so I can close my mouth. Where I get the strength, I don't know; except that prayer is certainly giving me strength.

I want to die alone; I am not afraid. I have seen the glory of heaven. Sorry I had to come back. Love, Ruth.

1-30-65   My voice comes back at night, and then I speak out loud. I don't want a neurologic examination. I can't stand hands touching me—I never could. I stiffen up. Last night I felt I was finished. A day of nausea and mucus. I stopped all medication; I am sick at the sight of one more pill. My stomach jumps up in horror. I need a rest from medication.

1-31-65   I am dying, slowly but surely. I need help and care. I can't stay with my employer, helping her; I am not up to it. I can't go on here. I can leave, and be alone till I die. At least no one will be blamed.

2-1-65   I feel better. I just got fighting mad. If I don't raise hell, I am as good as dead. I want to see you—you aways put my head back on straight. But I'll be damned if I need any strange doctors. I am either crazy or I'm getting well. You can be the best judge. I am resting, loafing, feeling better.

2-2-65   If I have nothing more, I have a fighting spirit; I just keep walking forward. I never look back.

2-4-65   Dear Dr. A., Dorothy and Carolyn; thank you for calling me. It's good, knowing that somewhere in this city I do not stand alone. My voice becomes normal when I have not eaten. I can laugh and smile now. I need FREE-

DOM now. The sooner I stand on two feet, the better. You know how I am—dying one minute, up the next. I am not worried about me. It's over.

2-6-65 Friday, my little finger on my right hand would not stand up; it hung down. Yesterday, both arms and hands were numb. It's amazing; I am making such a quick comeback. Yesterday I ate a sandwich. My speech is coming along, so I feel cheered up. Since I am not famous, when I go I won't be missed. I believe one should die in peace and dignity as God has given one the right to do.

I never knew taking a bath and washing my hair could be such a big job. But I am neat and clean. I am coming along, and am anxious to see all of you.

2-8-65 The time to be brave and fool myself is OVER. I need care, not work. I can't go on here. I am exhausted. I may have to ask United Charities to help me. I can't prepare food and eat it. If I live, it must be care now. It's time I am going now, not later. I have no family. I am not well; I won't be for a long time, and well I know it.

2-9-65 I feel better, and plan to get well. Don't worry if you don't hear from me. I want freedom from all medical care. I can't stand care. I gather laundry and I shop for food. I have been crying on everybody's shoulder long enough. It's time to stand up and fight. My hearing is very poor. Don't worry if you receive no letter. I look well. Getting mad won't kill me any sooner. But I am no doormat. I will earn money. I don't need help, and I should be paid. So I am sailing out again with my ship under control. I am now at peace. I can do all housework, except scrubbing floors.

2-19-65 Trying to hold a job I can't do is foolish; I need rest and care. As long as I can stand up and do some work, fine, but I can't eat. All the strength I gain can't last.

2-26-65 The social worker I called is going to look around for a home for me. I cannot go on the way I am now.

I don't plan to turn back—I need help. Whatever lies in the future, at least one door opened.

2-27-65 I am getting weaker; I can't swallow food. My appetite is gone.

2-28-65 I feel better today. I was able to swallow a little meat loaf. I am resting, and honestly trying to get well. I sleep fine. I had one seizure, early this morning and it relieved me a lot—I needed it. Please do not worry. God is watching over me, as you can see. It always makes me feel bad when I cause you any worry.

3-1-65 I have a strange feeling that your thoughts are with me. I have at last a sense of peace. God is with me. Here I can die. When it looks so dark, suddenly it is bright.

3-5-65 I am feeling stronger, resting quite a bit. My employer said I do not have to work; if I can prepare a meal, do dishes, iron, and take laundry down, that is fine; when I feel I can't, it is all right to say so.

I have been through a bad time. I had two days of double vision, and I seemed to walk in a dark cloud. That cleared up. Mucus is better. I am quiet, talking a little, clearly, occasionally. I walk around the house, lie down or sit up in a chair. But I rest and don't worry. Nothing I can do but ride out this storm quietly. When I left off taking medicine, I had seizures.

My eyes were so distorted, window shades zigzagged, pictures, all objects had two or four faces. It was really amusing. I am trying to get well. Being alive now, getting useful, doing a job, is most important.

3-7-65 Motion is returning to my face. I can whistle a little. I smile occasionally. I can blow my nose, which formerly I was not able to do. So all is clearing up. I am calm, relaxed. In all the years I have been your patient, when did God forget me?

Being independent helps me a lot.

3-18-65 Dr. Alvarez—the TRUTH please. Will I ever be able to swallow food in a normal manner? So far, all I can take is in liquid form. I am awakened at night occasionally with my throat filled. Can this be helped?

I get depressed, but that doesn't last; I cheer myself on. But I must decide my future. Can I be helped to live a normal life? I do not care how long it takes, I will keep on trying to get well.

3-25-65 The time to fool myself is OVER. I am exhausted. It's time I am going—now, not later.

[THAT WAS THE LAST LETTER I RECEIVED FROM RUTH. ON APRIL 1, 1965, SHE DIED, AND AT LAST SHE FOUND THE PEACE THAT SHE HAD CRAVED DURING MOST OF HER FIFTY-EIGHT MUCH-TROUBLED YEARS.]

L'Envoi

How wonderful it would be if Ruth could be here today to see her story of suffering all typed and in print. How proud she would feel, and how glad she would be that at last millions of people who are still suffering as she had so suffered, can get a hint as to what, for long, perhaps for all their days, has been ruining their health—a "dysrhythmic electroencephalogram"—and could almost overnight be relieved with the help of a wonderful medicine.

As Ruth knew so well, nearly all of the few million people in our country who are suffering terribly from a dysrhythmia are wasting thousands of dollars on ineffectual psychotherapy, many examinations, and perhaps one or two abdominal operations.

Ruth hoped that thousands of persons, on reading a few pages of this book, would say, "Why, that's me; those are my symptoms. Now I know what has been distressing me all my days." Immediately such a person should try to get electroencephalograms made, and especially if they show a dysrhythmia, or lack of normal rhythm, a doctor would do well to try the effect of an anti-convulsant drug.

Also, Ruth hoped that many of the people who were greatly helped by the drug would quickly pass on a word of hope to a number of people they knew who, for all their days, had been looked on as "just a bunch of nerves" with "nothing the matter."

For forty-eight years Ruth suffered untreated with mild epilepsy, never knowing the cause of her distress. Years of violent temper tantrums, blackouts, wild rages, uncontrollable anger, confusion, horrible nightmares and frightening hallucinations plagued her, and the only answer she could get from doctors was "It's just nerves."

Tranquilizers were not the solution; neither were sleep narcosis studies; stimulants didn't work. Then Ruth came to Dr. Walter C. Alvarez. Noticing slight muscle spasms, he prescribed Dilantin, a quieting, anti-convulsant drug. Dr. Alvarez diagnosed Ruth's symptoms as mild epilepsy—a form that induces no convulsions in its victims. And Dr. Alvarez, along with scores of other physicians, believes that for every case of convulsive epilepsy that is treated, far more cases of mild epilepsy are not detected, wrecking many lives. Dr. Alvarez estimates that there are several million mild epileptics in America today who do not know the cause of their miserable suffering.

So this is Ruth's story—what her life was like as a practicing nurse and then a housekeeper—how Dilantin affected her condition—how she lived and coped with and accepted her lot in life.

Ruth wrote to Dr. Alvarez for the last ten years of her life as a form of therapy and through a need during that time for self-purpose and a sense of usefulness. She trusted him and believed as he does that her story can benefit those many unfortunate people who do not know where to turn for help. As Dr. Alvarez writes, in his introduction to Ruth's story, "It certainly could bring health to a few million people if they could only read of her sufferings and say to themselves, 'Why, I have most of the symptoms that Ruth had.' Then they could take Dilantin, and perhaps be almost well overnight, as she became almost well."